CLIFF SHEATS'
LEAN BODIES

The Revolutionary New Approach to Losing Bodyfat

by Increasing Calories

CLIFF SHEATS

with Maggie Greenwood-Robinson

THE SUMMIT GROUP

FORT WORTH, TEXAS

THE SUGGESTIONS FOR SPECIFIC FOODS,
nutritional supplements, and exercise in this book are not intended
as a substitute for consultation with your physician.
After you have met your desired body composition goals, it is recommended
that you consult with a qualified health professional to establish food intake to
maintain your energy needs. Long-term usage of nutritional supplementation is not
recommended unless done so under the guidance of a physician, clinical
nutritionist, or registered dietician.
Individual dietary needs vary, and no diet or nutrition program will meet
everyone's daily requirements. Before starting the Lean Bodies program or an
exercise program, always see your physician. The use of specific products in this
book does not constitute an endorsement by the authors or the publisher.

THE SUMMIT GROUP
1227 West Magnolia, Suite 500, Fort Worth, Texas 76104

Printed in the United States of America

10   9   8

Library of Congress Catalog Card Number: 92-53772

LIBRARY OF CONGRESS CATALOGING IN PUBLICATION DATA

Sheats, Cliff.
    Cliff Sheats' lean bodies : the revolutionary new approach to losing bodyfat
by increasing calories / Cliff Sheats & Maggie Greenwood-Robinson ; introduction
by Bob Lanier.
        p. cm.
        Includes index.
        Includes recipes, sample menus, participating restaurants list, index
        ISBN 1-56530-007-6

        1. Nutrition. 2. Reducing diets. 3. Reducing diets – Recipes.
4. Reducing exercises. I. Greenwood-Robinson, Maggie. II. Title.
III. Title: The revolutionary new approach to losing bodyfat by increasing calories.

RM222.2.S53 1992   613.24
                     QB192-10283

To Kathy and Jonathan

Cliff Sheats' Lean Bodies

CONTEN

T S

vii   FOREWORD

ix   ACKNOWLEDGMENTS

xi   INTRODUCTION

xiii   LETTER TO THE SCIENTIFIC COMMUNITY

1   CHAPTER ONE   *It's Time to Eat!*

27   CHAPTER TWO   *Lean Protein: A Metabolic Activator*

43   CHAPTER THREE   *Carbohydrates: Fuel and Fiber*

57   CHAPTER FOUR   *EFAs and MCTs: The Healthy Fats*

69   CHAPTER FIVE   *A Leaner Body in Just Seven Weeks*

101   CHAPTER SIX   *Accelerating Bodyfat Loss*

109   CHAPTER SEVEN   *Vitamins: Metabolic Catalysts*

123   CHAPTER EIGHT   *Minerals and Other Amazing Nutrients*

139   CHAPTER NINE   *Fat-Burning / Health-Building Exercise*

169   CHAPTER TEN   *Nutritional Needs of Exercisers and Athletes*

185   CHAPTER ELEVEN   *Leaner and Fitter For a Lifetime*

197   NOTES   *References*

205   APPENDIX A   *Questions and Answers About Lean Bodies*

217   APPENDIX B   *Lean Bodies Cooking*

263   APPENDIX C   *Recommended Products*

267   APPENDIX D   *Food Composition Guide*

283   APPENDIX E   *Participating Lean Bodies Restaurants*

295   GLOSSARY

307   INDEX

Foreword

A VERY FRUSTRATING PART of medical practice is watching patients who try to lose weight and fail. The doctor and the patient both feel like failures and they often give up simultaneously. The weight is then an unmentionable in subsequent visits. Unfortunately, this is all too common in American society.

Take Jack S. who has been coming to me for years. His weight will fluctuate as much as 40 pounds in a twelve-month period. In spite of his best efforts, his weight is never close to ideal. He has tried every diet conceived and every mode of exercising you can imagine. He is certainly motivated. Many Americans are just like this. They may be less motivated but, like Jack, their hope is eternal.

That's why I'm so pleased about Cliff's new book. The Lean Bodies program is a safe, effective method of controlling weight and total bodyfat. This program is not a diet. It is a lifetime change in eating habits. I believe it is an effective program, and I recommend it to patients daily. If you have trouble with your weight, I recommend it to you also. As a physician, I'm so gratified to see my patients on a plan that works, and this one really does. Try the Lean Bodies program, and turn your own diet failures into long-term success.

Jack E. Ireland, M.D., Family Practitioner

Acknowledgments

WRITING A BOOK brings together many people, with many contributions. Consequently, there are many to thank – for without them, there would be no book. First, I would like to thank my wife Kathy for her encouragement and enduring love. During the inevitable ups and downs in life, she never faltered, and that is why she has the affection of my heart; also, my son Jonathan for his patience with "Dat" while I was finishing this project. Next, I thank my parents, my brother and sister, as well as my in-laws, for believing in me and giving me the encouragement to pursue my goals.

I would like to express my appreciation to my staff for going beyond "the call of duty" to help make this book a reality.

I am indebted to my friend and colleague John Parrillo of Cincinnati, Ohio, who pioneered the high-calorie approach to eating by working with elite athletes for the past 20 years. Where nutrition is concerned, John is light years ahead of the pack, and I have benefited greatly from his knowledge and experience. Thank you, John, also for reviewing the manuscript and for lending your discerning eye to its contents.

I am not sure that there would even be a Lean Bodies without Larry North, the host of "The Weekend Workout" on KLIF and the owner of North Bodies, a fitness center in Dallas. Through the enormous reach of KLIF, Larry has spread the word about Lean Bodies and has been one of its strongest advocates. Larry also gave me the opportunity to be the resident nutritionist – and frequent co-host – on his show. That opportunity has meant everything to me, and I remain forever grateful.

I would also like to thank Roland Jehl, the owner of The Austin Gym in Dallas, for his advice and for his confidence in the program.

My deep thanks go to clinical nutritionist Luke Bucci, Ph.D., an inspiration to me in my profession. Dr. Bucci is a cutting edge professional, and his work in performance nutrition stands second to none. Dr. Bucci, thank you for taking time out of your busy schedule to review the manuscript and give us your comments and suggestions.

My thanks are also extended to Jack Ireland, M.D., for his support of my program in regard to public health awareness and to Bob Lanier, M.D., for his encouragement and foresight.

My special thanks go to C.T. Smith, Ph.D., and J.A. Gilbertson-Smith, Ph.D., of The American Council of Applied Clinical Nutrition for equipping me with the tools of my profession – and to my friend Lucia Dubose, Ph.D., for sharing with me her wealth of knowledge in the field of nutrition. I am also grateful to my friend Dr. William Cowden, M.D., for all his support and encouragement during my early years as a clinical nutritionist. My warmest regards are extended to all of my associates in The International and American Association of Clinical Nutritionists for helping put the science of nutrition on the map.

I know for certain that there would not be a book without my co-author Maggie Greenwood-Robinson. Maggie organized the program into a superbly written, easy-to-follow format. In addition, she committed to one of the tightest book writing schedules on record and did it in the collaborative, enthusiastic spirit for which she is known. She is, in my opinion, one of the most talented and creative individuals in her field. I am also very grateful to Jeff Robinson for his technical services on the project.

Another special note of appreciation goes to Linda Thornbrugh for her "art of cooking" techniques and exceptional organizational skills.

My thanks and appreciation also go to all the "lean bodies" who have been through my classes for proving that you can lose bodyfat by increasing calories and for starting the revolution in the way America diets.

Next, I thank my publisher, The Summit Group, for believing in this project, pouring their energies into every single aspect of it, and making the dream of it come true. Like everyone else involved in this project, Summit knew that the time was right for this revolution.

Ultimately, this entire program would not be possible without the sovereign direction of my Heavenly Father.

Cliff Sheats
Dallas, Texas

Introduction

EVERY YEAR AROUND CHRISTMAS I designate a big box on the floor by my desk as the "diet-book" box. By February each year it bulges and flows over as publishing houses freely send me the new year's crop hoping I will publicize them on my radio and television syndication. Fat chance. For the most part diet books are like fruit-cakes. There's really just one; they keep changing the name and passing it around the next year. I've become pretty cynical. About the only time I mention diet books now is to poke fun at them, and it's usually pretty easy to do.

But then I heard a young fellow on a local radio show one morning about two years ago who seemed to have come up with a genuinely unique approach. He said you didn't have to starve yourself; in fact, if you ate more you could weigh less. It was a little like having a banker tell you the way to make your savings grow is to spend more. I was intrigued and began to make it a point to listen regularly. I finally called Cliff Sheats and asked for his book. To my surprise, he didn't have one. And to his surprise, he found a lot of people like me who wanted one. And that's the origin of Lean Bodies. It was "written on request."

The remarkable concept Cliff presents is that weight control should not be a program of punishing exercise combined with starvation. We've all done that routine, and we've all failed. Those painful episodes do not have any long-lasting effect other than to make the body more resistant to weight loss in the future. Indeed, doctors are many times a little less than enthusiastic about dieting because we almost always see people put the weight back on. We'll tell you to lose weight but we don't like you to look us in the eye and say, "What is the realistic chance I can do it?" You don't want to know.

In Lean Bodies, Cliff Sheats gives doctors a reason to be enthusiastic about weight control again. He adds the dimension of "increasing the metabolism" which allows people to lose weight with moderate exercise while eating more. Lean

Bodies may not be the last word in diet books, but it offers more promise than anything I've seen in years.

Dr. Bob Lanier, M.D.,
Host of TV's "60-Second Housecall"

Letter to the Scientific Community

YES, EVEN SCIENTISTS have the "herd" instinct. When I first heard of the concept of eating more to control weight, I, like most scientists, was skeptical. After all, food deprivation does cause weight loss. A "normal" weight could then be maintained by never consuming more than the number of calories expended each day. This approach seemed to work well. Supportive studies were published and quickly embraced by the medical and dietary communities.

With the passage of time, however, this approach did not have universal application. Some people still manage to gain weight at caloric intakes that should have starved them. Others fell into the classic "yo-yo" dieting cycles of weight loss, followed by ever-greater weight gain. Other people did well but were terribly frustrated at not being able to eat their favorite foods or maintain their eating program while dining out.

Unfortunately, a major experimental variable — the ability of a person's metabolic rate to change in response to both quantity and quality of food intake levels — was seldom examined. We do know that metabolic rates will change in response to varying food intake: Less food yields a lower metabolic rate, which results in fewer calories needed to maintain weight. With this pattern, chronic dieters, especially victims of the yo-yo dieting cycles, down-regulated their metabolic rates lower than previously calculated tables of data for their height, weight, and other measurable variables.

Clearly, another approach was needed to address the long-term goal of healthy weight normalization. Enter sports nutrition. For years, strength athletes have consumed far more calories and protein than their sedentary counterparts but remained leaner and more muscular. The difference in body appearance was attributed to a greater number of calories expended by athletes during exercise. Later, exercise was shown to stimulate metabolic rate beyond the additional caloric demands of exertion alone. Thus, athletes could consume 5,000 calories a day or more and still remain fit and trim.

Finally, the simple question was asked: If people can down-regulate metabolic rate by eating fewer calories, can eating more calories up-regulate metabolic rate? It turns out that the answer is yes, but certain conditions apply. These involve research-based understandings of lipid metabolism, micro-nutrient status, food/insulin interaction, and the proper ratio of protein, carbohydrates and fats in the diet.

Application of this latest research has resulted in a common sense, scientific approach to reducing bodyfat in a healthy and energy-producing matter — the Lean Bodies program. Lean Bodies addresses the diet and exercise conditions necessary to increase caloric intake to up-regulate metabolism in a reproducible and individual manner.

At a time when many healthcare professionals and scientists are following the "herd" instinct of fewer calories/less weight, I congratulate Cliff Sheats for successfully applying the concept of more calories, less bodyfat.

Dr. Luke R. Bucci, Ph.D., C.C.N.
Biochemist, Innerpath Nutrition

Dr. Bucci is the Director of Science and Quality for SpectraCell Laboratories in Houston, Texas, a new diagnostic clinical lab introducing a functional essay for nutritional status. Dr. Bucci is also a Certified Clinical Nutritionist at InnerPath Nutrition, specializing in advanced nutritional counseling and education. Dr. Bucci is the author of "Nutrients As Ergogenic Aids in Sport and Exercise" by the CRC Press, teaches nutrition and physiology classes for college students, gives relicensing seminars on nutrition for healthcare professionals, and consults for home healthcare companies. Dr. Bucci received his Ph.D. in Biochemistry at the University of Texas at Houston Graduate School of Biomedical Sciences. After a postdoctoral appointment in cancer research at M.D. Anderson Hospital in Houston, he served as Research Director for a nutritional supplement company.

1

❚ *It's Time to Eat!*

AMERICA HAS GONE HUNGRY LONG ENOUGH. We have been duped by diet gurus into self-imposed starvation. We have tried fasting, liquid diets, laxative abuse — even stomach stapling and intestinal bypasses. But all of these, no matter how dramatic, are just extreme forms of that mainstay of American dieting, cutting calories. This has all gone far enough. It's painful, it's health destroying, and it doesn't even work.

What *does* work is *increasing calories to lose bodyfat*. That is right. Increasing. I know that some of you reading this will not believe it; our society has been completely brainwashed into accepting low-calorie diets as the only way to lose weight. But ten years from now, this revolutionary approach to losing bodyfat will be accepted absolutely and without question, and Americans will look back and wonder why they ever bought into the low-calorie approach.

Eating to lose bodyfat — it sounds too good to be true! Yet, not only is it true, it is the *only* way to successfully lose bodyfat and keep it off. On the new Lean Bodies program, you can and will lose bodyfat by increasing calories — to 1,800, 2,500, even 3,600 calories a day — all while you get leaner and fitter than you have ever been in your life. No more starving yourself, no more regaining all the weight you worked so hard to lose.

This program, which truly is revolutionary, will dramatically speed up your metabolism and turn your body into a highly efficient fat burner. You will notice the changes almost immediately, and you get measurable results in just seven weeks. And after seven weeks, this program offers you a lifestyle you can maintain and enjoy easily.

What Is Lean Bodies?

Let me tell you a little bit about how Lean Bodies came to be. In the late 1980s, while working with a cardiologist and in private practice, I designed a revolutionary new fat loss method. This new approach to fat loss, called the Lean Bodies program, is based on the very latest research in nutrition and human metabolism.

In my practice, I have worked with people who had a range of problems, including obesity, high blood pressure, high cholesterol, diabetes, hypoglycemia, and chronic fatigue. Even though their problems were different, they had two things in common: First, they were not eating enough food to fuel their bodies efficiently. Second, what little food they did eat was the wrong kind. But the latest research shows that losing bodyfat depends on eating *more* calories, not fewer. Further research shows that the body's ability to build muscle depends less on exercise and more on eating habits than was previously thought. In my opinion, 75 percent of the body's ability to gain lean mass is a matter of nutrition.

Clearly, American eating habits *have* to change. So I created an optimal nutritional plan called Lean Bodies. It started modestly and then grew to become one of the most successful fat loss programs in North Texas. Now it is available for the first time in book form to everyone across the nation.

Permission to Eat

In modern American society, far too many people try to live on the smallest amount of food possible — and they put their health on the line as a result. In the Lean Bodies classes, we call this practice "self-inflicted" starvation, and, sadly, many people subject themselves to this torture for years. They never realize that the human body *needs* food – specific, healthy kinds of food. My own experience with poor nutrition taught me this lesson and began my lifelong interest in the subject.

I entered the field of nutrition because it restored my health when I was much younger. In college, I was playing on the tennis team, and we would eat chocolate candy bars so that we could play longer. As a result, I got in the habit of eating candy – even to the point of substituting sugar for meals to keep my energy up. Eventually, I started feeling tired and weak all the time. My sugar "addiction" had erupted into full-blown hypoglycemia. Severe allergies followed, and it became difficult to breathe or do much of anything.

To treat the allergies, I was put on various medications – so many in fact that I had to carry them around with me all day. I stuffed them in my tennis racket cover, and it bulged with bottles and jars. Needless to say, the medication only aggravated my already failing health. This went on for a few years, until a friend at church told me about a Dr. Marshall Ringsdorf.

Desperate, I went to see him. He took one look at my blood tests and told me my problems could all be corrected with nutrition. I was floored! Dr. Ringsdorf took me off medication and put me on a high protein, high complex carbohydrate, high calorie diet, along with nutritional supplements. In two weeks, I felt so good that I decided to run. I ran around the block, then stopped for a moment to see if I was all right. The feeling of having regained my strength was so overwhelming that I was overcome with emotion.

I started playing tennis again (one doctor had told me to give it up). And nine months later I was playing on a professional tennis circuit against world class athletes.

A while later, I had a complete physical, and I'll never forget what the doctor said: "There's no place to rate you on our scale. You're above 'excellent.' In fact, you are in the superior range."

As a result of these and other experiences, I decided to pursue a career in nutrition. I realize now that I had to endure my early health problems to better understand what others are going through – and to recognize how vital food is to good health.

That is why the Lean Bodies program stresses food – plenty of food, healthy food, and good food. On this program you will enjoy things like Herbed Potato Skins, Savory Poultry Strips, Barbecued Shrimp, and Sauteed New Potatoes. You will find these and many more in Appendix B. In addition, the *Lean Bodies Cookbook* is currently available.

On the Lean Bodies program, you rediscover the importance of food for achieving optimum health and fitness. You will see that food is really fuel – fuel for a high energy, healthy lifestyle. And you'll enjoy really good food, not tiny portions or liquid meals.

Starvation Does Not Work Anyway

All of the calorie-cutting approaches America is so fascinated with are really a threat to good health, and, to top it off, they don't even work.

An example is Ed H., a telecommunications engineer, who is one of our many inspiring Lean Bodies cases.

Ed had been fat all his life. When he was a child, kids called him "fat boy" to his face. As he grew to manhood, he was still called "fat boy," but behind his back.

At age 35, Ed made up his mind to lose weight. With that decision began a long and tortuous history of dieting, starting with organized weight loss groups. One group emphasized liver in its food plan, and

Ed developed gout as a result. He dropped in and out of various weight-loss groups until finally deciding on a last-ditch effort to get thin: the intestinal bypass, a procedure touted in the seventies as a viable weight-loss alternative. A five-year case of diarrhea, not weight loss, was his reward.

From there, Ed ran the gamut of dieting, from the grapefruit diet to the boiled egg diet. Like many dieters, he finally resorted to a medically-supervised liquid fast. He lost 15 pounds but gained cold sores and boils in his mouth during the fast. Meanwhile, Ed got uric acid stones as a result of his intestinal bypass. He had to take Demerol to ease the pain of passing the stones and then got hooked on the drug.

His next move was to have the intestinal operation reversed. The surgery caused a bowel impaction, and he almost died.

Upon his wife's urging, Ed came to Lean Bodies. He had reached an all-time high of 316 pounds. After 23 weeks on the program, he weighed in at 252. Ed eats 5,000 calories a day and is still losing bodyfat.

As Ed's early diet history so poignantly shows, you're endangering your health by dieting. Judy I., who lost 35 pounds on the program, puts it this way: "I feel guilty if I don't eat. It used to be the other way around."

Weight Versus Fat

While following the Lean Bodies program, you focus primarily on losing bodyfat rather than on losing weight. The terms "weight" and "fat" are often used interchangeably, but they are really quite different. "Weight" is a measurement that includes the combined weight of muscle, fat, body fluids, organs, skin, and bones. "Fat" refers to one of three types of tissue: subcutaneous fat, which is found directly under the skin; stored fat, which is usually deposited around the hips, thighs, or abdomen; and essential fat, which envelops, protects, and cushions cellular membranes, nerves, and vital organs. Losing bodyfat means losing stored fat — the flab that makes you look out of shape and unhealthy.

Occasionally, people on my program have a difficult time weaning themselves from the scales. Cheryl Y., an on-and-off dieter for years as well as a former diet pill user, at first felt "depressed because the needle on the scale wasn't moving to the left." But then Cheryl discovered that she had lost nearly five percent of her bodyfat — a considerable loss and one that made noticeable changes in her figure.

"When I lost weight on diet pills, I got skinny but I was never firm," she says. "By losing bodyfat, I now look firmer and harder than I have in years."

In the Lean Bodies program, we speak a slightly different language than other diet programs do. For example, we talk "bodyfat percentage" in addition to pounds lost. You will say "I dropped from 27 percent bodyfat to 15 percent." We also talk "lean mass." This refers to the amount of muscle you're carrying. Muscle is important because it's the body's most metabolically active tissue. The more lean mass you carry, the faster your metabolism. Incidentally, muscle alone weighs two and a half times more than fat, so concentrating on how much you "weigh" gives you an imprecise reading of how much bodyfat you're actually carrying.

Before starting the program, it's important to understand what the desirable percentages of bodyfat are:

Well-conditioned men: under 12 percent

Normally active men: 13 to 16 percent

Well-conditioned women: under 18 percent

Normally active women: 19 to 24 percent

These ranges should help you set your goals for bodyfat loss. In

Chapter 5, I explain how to obtain an accurate measurement of bodyfat.

What To Expect

The Lean Bodies program teaches you to eat to lose your bodyfat, without cutting calories or resorting to a starvation-type diet. In fact, this program isn't a "diet" at all. It's an effective, nutritionally-based eating program for losing bodyfat and keeping it off forever.

Once you start following this program, you'll discover how to:

• Accelerate your metabolism to burn fat.

• Boost your energy level far beyond what you've ever experienced.

• Eat correctly to maintain your desired weight for a lifetime.

• Understand the often-complicated subject of nutrition so you can learn to think for yourself.

• Feel more self-confident and healthier than you ever have.

Meet Some Lean Bodies

Thousands of people just like you have followed my program and experienced remarkable success. They've lost bodyfat – and have kept it off. They feel energetic for the first time in years. They've overcome certain health problems, such as high cholesterol and low blood sugar.

Many of the people who follow the Lean Bodies program have been "yo-yo" dieters, going on and off diets and up and down in weight. Sue L., for example, started the program weighing 162 pounds. She ate all the wrong foods and resorted to diet shakes to lose weight. Not only that, she was a "couch potato" and had very little energy.

"After six weeks on Cliff's program," she says, "I lost 25 pounds and 5 percent bodyfat and was eating more food than I had in years and losing weight. Overall, I lost a total of 31 pounds and 12 percent bodyfat. I just love a program that lets you eat to lose bodyfat."

My Lean Bodies classes are filled with liquid diet "dropouts" — people who have followed medically-supervised fasts. In most cases, they have regained their weight or are well on their way to doing so. Some have even become quite ill after following this starvation-like regimen.

Gene H. calls those diets "misery." After losing 60 pounds on a liquid diet, he was afraid he would gain it all back. Wanting to keep his weight off for good, Gene started the Lean Bodies classes and learned how to eat again — and keep his bodyfat off.

"I went from 25 percent bodyfat to 16 percent bodyfat. Now I don't care about what I weigh anymore. The important thing is how I look and how my clothes fit.

"Since I've been on Cliff's program, people kid me about having the face of a 55-year-old and the body of a 25-year-old."

Mike M. is another liquid diet dropout. Repetitive dieting, including liquid diets, ultimately sent his weight zooming (345 pounds with a bodyfat measurement of 50 percent) and his energy plummeting. Mike was shocked when he saw a picture of himself taken at a birthday party. At first, he didn't recognize the portly figure in the picture. When reality set in, he decided to do something about it.

Over several months, Mike gradually upped his calories to 7,000 a day, while starting a walking program and a regular routine of weight training. In just four months, he dropped his weight to 255 and his bodyfat to 27 percent. Mike is so enthused about his results that he wants to become a personal trainer to others with weight problems.

Driven to get thin, some people resort to a lifetime of dangerous dieting habits. Robbie W. is a good example. She had been a chubby child and teenager. While she was in high school, her family internist suggested that she take diet pills for 30 days. Robbie followed his advice and lost 30 pounds. She vowed never to be fat again, and for the next four years she kept that vow. Later, however, her weight began to creep back up again. For the next several years, she took prescription diet pills off and on while receiving diuretic injections. Except during her pregnancy at age 23, Robbie was on diet pills for the next 15 years.

Finally, the diet pills took their toll. Two years ago, medical tests confirmed that she had a heart condition exacerbated by diet pills and decongestants. She stopped taking both, and her weight shot up. In desperation, she cut her calories back to about 800 a day and began exercising six days a week.

"To my frustration, I actually gained weight," Robbie says. "My metabolism had finally shut down. I got in touch with Cliff and started his program. It was a miracle and a life saver. Today, I'm 20 pounds lighter. I dropped from 30-percent bodyfat to 24-percent bodyfat. I eat 2,500 calories a day, and I feel wonderful."

Not everyone who starts the Lean Bodies program wants to lose bodyfat. Many want to gain lean mass (muscle). Gary D., for example, was like a human stick figure, standing six feet tall and weighing a mere 150 pounds. Although he had lifted weights for several years, he was never able to significantly increase his body weight. Following the program, Gary boosted his calories up to 3,500 a day. In only four months, he gained 18 pounds of lean mass while keeping his bodyfat at a healthy 10.5 percent.

"I now understand that the formula for gaining lean mass is 75 percent nutrition and 25 percent exercise," he says. "Thanks to this eating program, I'm still gaining."

Have you ever noticed how tired you feel when you're dieting? Fatigue sets in when you're not fueling your body with enough calories and nutrients to keep it going. You feel chronically de-energized as a result.

After just two weeks on the Lean Bodies program, Donna J. noticed she had more energy than ever. At the same time, she was losing bodyfat. By following the program, she was able to reduce her bodyfat from 26 percent to a healthy, lean 19 percent. "Lean Bodies made a big difference in my life," she says.

A chronic lack of physical and mental energy spurred Ira A. to try the program. He was employed in a high stress job that required him to travel more than 200,000 air miles every year. Almost every day, he would feel so weary and dragged out that he had to take a nap.

Ira stuck to the program religiously, weaning himself from coffee and sugary foods and learning to eat the right foods in proper amounts and combinations. At first, his fatigue made it difficult for him to exercise, but he persevered nonetheless. After 18 months, he was walking a brisk three miles a day, lifting weights, and playing on a men's baseball team. He shed the 15 pounds he wanted to lose. And no longer does he take afternoon naps.

The Lean Bodies program works for people of all ages. Lynn B. was an overweight 16-year-old high school student. Like most people, he had tried every diet and lost weight – only to gain it back. "I thought you had to starve yourself to get thin," he says. Faced with the prospect of staying fat the rest of his life, Lynn came to Lean Bodies for help. As a result, he lost 44 pounds and gained 15 pounds of lean mass.

"Diets fail because they starve the body. Cliff's program fuels the body. I'm so glad I went to Cliff's program. It has really changed my life."

Physicians refer their patients to my program for a variety of reasons, in addition to fat loss. Diabetics, for example, find that the program helps stabilize their blood sugar. Linda P. has been a type-II diabetic for more than two years. Prior to beginning the program, she drank fruit juice in response to insulin reactions – only to experience uncomfortable highs. Now, instead of fruit juice, she drinks the protein/carbohydrate supplement recommended by the Lean Bodies program, which doesn't cause a sugar high.

"It stabilizes my blood sugar, and I no longer have the highs. I feel healthier than ever."

My program is a low-fat, nutrient-rich eating plan, and that's the reason people can regain their health by following it. Gaylene E. is a good example. Just before she started the program, she had a blood test, and it registered her total cholesterol at 240.*

With the help of the program, she has been able to reduce her cholesterol significantly. She also lost four inches around her waist and a total of 11 pounds.

"I have more lean mass, and I have energy left over – and that's a first for me! I think Cliff's program will guarantee any change in your body that you want!"

Donna T. was facing the possibility of a stroke at age 47, according to her neurologist. She was diagnosed as having clogged arteries and high cholesterol (268) as well as being a borderline diabetic. In addition, Donna suffered from severe migraine headaches, for which she took medication that caused a lot of unpleasant side effects.

As Donna tells it: "Naturally, I was scared by my prognosis. I was too young for my children to take care of me." Donna's brother-in-law, who was already on the Lean Bodies program, suggested that she give it try, and she did. After 30 days on the program, her cholesterol dropped to 226, and she was able to go off her headache medication completely. "My doctor was floored."

---

*A healthy total cholesterol reading is typically below 200. Between 200 and 239 is considered borderline, and above 239 is considered a risk factor for heart disease.

Plus, Donna was able to shed 16 pounds, including a "few rolls around my waistline."

Never Say Diet Again

If you're like most dieters, you've probably lost and regained hundreds of pounds in your lifetime – and you've done it by restricting calories.

In theory, restricting calories to lose bodyfat sounds like a good idea, but in reality, this approach simply doesn't work. That's because low-calorie diets are really a form of starvation. Yes, you lose weight initially but only because the body is eating itself – its own tissue, muscles, and organs – to maintain life. This process is physically destructive. Parts of your body are dying.

When you go on a low-calorie diet, very little of what you lose is bodyfat. I once consulted with a man who had been following a liquid shake diet. He would drink his shakes during the day and eat a meal at night. After two and a half weeks, he had lost approximately 10 pounds. An analysis of his body composition (the ratio of muscle to bodyfat), however, revealed that he had lost mostly muscle tissue and very little bodyfat! His body had turned into a cannibal, feeding on its own muscle tissue to survive.

Losing muscle tissue in this manner can be debilitating. Dr. Chuck A., a physician who completed my program, told me about his father, Dr. Chuck A., Sr., who had contracted a neuromuscular disease called polymyositis that results in an irreversible deterioration of voluntary muscle tissue. This condition was caused by repeated low-calorie dieting.

Upon his son's urging, Chuck Sr. started my program. After six weeks, medical tests found a slowing of muscle deterioration. Although Chuck Sr.'s condition is chronic, his quality of life has been greatly improved by proper nutrition, including increased calories.

Low-calorie diets also slow your metabolism, the physiological process that converts food to energy so that your body can run. A sluggish metabolism means that your body cannot burn calories efficiently. As a result, the excess calories are stored as fat. Unless you start eating to restore your metabolism, it will remain sluggish.

In addition, research shows that your metabolic rate drops considerably following a period of caloric restriction. A study published in The American Journal of Clinical Nutrition compared the metabolic rates of two groups: 16 women who had lost weight by following a low-calorie diet and 16 women who were already lean with no history of weight problems. Both groups had similar body composition measurements (the ratio of muscle to bodyfat). The study found that the first group (the dieters who had lost weight) had metabolic rates that were 15 percent lower than the other group of women.[1]

Every time you diet and then go off it, it becomes harder for you to lose weight the next time you diet. That's the conclusion of research done in both animals and humans. In one study of 1,000 obese patients who were put on weight-loss programs between 1973 and 1983, researchers found that the rate of weight loss slowed with successive diets. They stated in the study that "chronic dieting may lead to permanent metabolic and physiological alterations which promote weight gain and make subsequent loss of weight more difficult."[2]

There are many theories as to why this happens. One is that once you start eating normally again, your body accelerates its build-up of fat as if to prepare for the next "famine" (another diet). This famine/fat acceleration cycle makes you regain more bodyfat after each period of dieting.

Other factors are at work to keep you fat as well. Did you know, for example, that by not eating, you are training your body to store fat? Here's why: Your body contains an enzyme called lipoprotein lipase or LPL. Found on the surface of fat tissue, LPL governs fat storage. When you go on and off diets, your body starts producing more LPL – which in turn steps up fat production and storage.

Repetitive low-calorie dieting has many other severe consequences on health. For example:

• Studies show that when people regain pounds after dieting, blood pressure rises, and blood levels of glucose (blood sugar) and triglycerides (blood fats) increase.[3]

• Weight fluctuation ("yo-yo dieting") has been linked to heart disease – especially among men and women between the ages 30 to 44 – the age group in which dieting is the most common, according to an analysis of data from participants in the Framingham Heart Study.* The risk factors for coronary heart disease in this age group (30 to 44) were comparable to coronary risk factors associated with obesity! That's frightening, especially if you consider the fact that about 50 percent of American women and 25 percent of American men are on diets at any given time – and most of the time, these diets fail.[4]

• When you lose and regain weight quickly, you're at risk for developing gallbladder disease. A study published in the Archives of Internal Medicine showed that 13 of 38 obese women and 13 obese men on a rapid weight loss program developed gallstones within eight weeks. All but one recovered after eating normal foods again.[5]

• The action of important digestive juices is diminished with low-calorie diets. When normal eating resumes, you start experiencing gas and are unable to handle certain foods.

• Overweight patients who go on low-calorie diets of between

---

*The Framingham Heart Study is a study of the health status of 5,127 men and women from Framingham, Massachusetts, who were initially free of coronary heart disease. Since 1948, their health has been monitored. The study cited above is based on data from 32 years of follow-up.

400 and 800 calories a day experience side effects that include fatigue, muscle cramps, headaches, hair loss, menstrual irregularities, and intolerance to cold.[6]

• Low-calorie diets not only cut calories, they also cut vital nutrients, such as protein, carbohydrates, essential fats, vitamins, and minerals. These are your "armed forces" for good health. When in short supply, these nutrients cannot adequately defend your body against invaders. Your immune system is weakened as a result, and you're a target for disease.

• Some diets can kill. In the late 1960s and early 1970s, the first "very-low-calorie diets" were introduced, and these took the form of powdered formulas mixed in water. The diets supplied about 400 calories a day. They were so popular that more such products were developed. In 1976, a best-selling diet book led to the widespread use of liquid protein products that were available over the counter. By the end of 1977, thousands of people had gone on this diet. As reported to the Centers for Disease Control, 60 people died as a result of ventricular arrhythmias (irregular heartbeat). The liquid protein diet was implicated as the cause of the heart problems.[7]

Even though liquid protein diets are off the market, liquid very-low-calorie meals are still with us. In connection with one particular brand that was popular several years ago, six deaths were reported. My contention is that these regimens are very damaging to health — and obviously life-threatening — because of their dangerously low level of calories and their questionable nutrient content. In fact, the primary ingredient in current formulations is sugar.

Unlike other diets, the Lean Bodies program is not nutrient-deficient. Nor is it a fad diet or any other quick fix. It is a sensible, effective, complete nutrition program that restores your metabolism, helps you lose bodyfat, and enables you to increase your health.

Dangerous Dieting

Our society puts a premium on looking good and being thin, and that's one reason why people try to lose weight fast – and at almost any cost. I have always been amazed and alarmed by the lengths to which people will go to lose weight. By itself, low-calorie dieting is danger-ous enough. But it's not the only unhealthy method used. Others include vomiting, fasting, diet drugs, laxatives, diuretics, and exces-sive exercise. All have serious health consequences, and it's important to understand the risks:[8]

Vomiting. Repeated, self-induced vomiting can cause a loss of potassium, a mineral vital for the healthy functioning of the heart and other muscles. Dizziness, weakness, low blood pressure, and tooth enamel erosion can also result.

Fasting. This is a severe and drastic measure for losing weight. Fasting causes rapid weight loss, but most of it is water and muscle tissue. Fasting also leads to serious nutritional deficiencies.

Diet drugs. To date, there's no magic pill to safely take off pounds. Although some drugs are used for weight control, the risks greatly outweigh the benefits. Amphetamines are stimulants that suppress the appetite. Dangerous and highly addictive, these drugs can cause gastrointestinal complications, restlessness, sleep problems, rapid heart rate, and even circulatory collapse. Your body quickly builds up a tolerance to amphetamines, so you have to take increasingly larger doses to feel the effects of the drug.

Because they accelerate the metabolic rate, thyroid hormones have been used to promote weight loss. The side effects of thyroid hormones, which include protein loss and heart complications, make these drugs an unwise and unsafe method of weight control.

Bulking agents are over-the-counter medications made with undigestible ingredients, usually methylcellulose and guar gum. When taken, they are supposed to create a feeling of fullness in the stomach, thereby suppressing the appetite. But health professionals warn that these products are ineffective and can cause intestinal gas.

Laxatives. Laxative abuse damages the nerves responsible for the colonic contractions that move waste products out of the body. The colon becomes immobilized while the laxatives do all the work. In time, not even laxatives will work, and enemas may have to be used. Even then, restoration of normal colonic functioning can take a while. Laxative abuse can also cause potassium depletion.

Diuretics. These are drugs that rid the body of fluids, resulting in water weight loss, which gives dieters a false sense of security when they weigh themselves. Excessive use of diuretics can cause muscular cramps, loss of vital minerals (including potassium), and heart rhythm problems, among other serious complications.

Excessive exercise. The desire to lose weight and the fear of gaining weight drive some people to extremes with exercise, often resulting in physical and psychological complications. These individuals exercise to the point of obsession, neglecting family life, social activities, and, ironically, personal health.

An article on runners in *The New England Journal of Medicine* described a man whose life had become so consumed with running that he cared about little else. He took up jogging after his daughter teased him about his paunch. Eventually, he began to run about 10 miles every day, without regard to weather or to the state of his health. He suffered from Achilles tendinitis and a slight limp brought on by a stress fracture that had not healed properly. He also liked to tally up the speed of each mile he ran and to take regular measurements of his lean body mass. Even though he was married, his relationship with his wife was cold and without sex.[9]

This case illustrates some of the psychological effects of excessive exercise: denial of pain, preoccupation with the activity, and social isolation. Equally important are the physical consequences. Exhaustion and fatigue, muscular strain, recurrent orthopedic injuries, and amenorrhea in women (the loss of monthly periods caused by extremely low levels of bodyfat) – these are all serious physical problems that can result from excessive exercise.

In the quest to lose weight, you can actually get hooked on health-threatening behaviors such as vomiting, excessive exercise, and laxative or diet drug abuse. Addiction to some of these behaviors can erupt in a full-blown eating disorder such as anorexia nervosa or bulimia. In fact, I believe that the biggest reasons for the rise of eating disorders are dieting and the dangerous dieting practices that go along with it.

Hopefully, with the introduction of the Lean Bodies program, I can persuade people that the healthiest way – and really the only way – to lose bodyfat is by increasing calories.

Changing Your Biochemistry

In the Lean Bodies program, I use the phrase "change your biochemistry." Simply put, this means speeding up your metabolism so that your body utilizes food more efficiently and burns bodyfat in the process. On this program, you can change your biochemistry by following four simple principles: gradually increase your calories, spread your calories throughout the day, choose metabolic-activating foods, and follow a program of moderate aerobic exercise.

Principle #1: Gradually increase your calories.

As I've mentioned, decreasing calories slows the metabolism, making it difficult for your body to burn fat. On this program, you gradually increase your calories, starting from a base and adding a certain number of calories each week. You burn bodyfat as a result.

If you're unconvinced, take the case of Paul, one of my clients in Dallas. Like many of the people I work with, Paul had tried practically every diet, including a medically-supervised liquid fast. On that particular program, he lost nearly 100 pounds but regained it in a few months.

With the goal of losing 90 pounds, Paul entered our program in February 1990. At the time, he weighed 281 pounds, and his bodyfat measured 30 percent. His metabolism was so sluggish that a daily caloric intake of 1,200 to 1,400 calories resulted in a weight gain. On the Lean Bodies program, he gradually increased his calories to 3,600 a day.

Between February and July 1990, Paul lost 86 pounds – and very little of this weight loss was muscle tissue. Remarkably, his bodyfat percentage dropped from 30 percent to a very healthy range. As Paul's case so clearly shows, adequate intake of calories boosts the metabolism for a fat-burning effect.

As you increase your calories, at first you'll feel as though you're force-feeding yourself. In truth though, you're training your metabolism to become more efficient – much like a novice runner would train himself to run faster and farther every time he hits the road. At first, he's so sluggish, he can barely run around the block. After adding a mile or two each day, he's at the head of the pack on race day. Your metabolism is no different. By gradually increasing calories, you kick your metabolism into high gear. You burn fat with a faster metabolism.

How will you know when your metabolism is faster? Here are the signs:

• You're eating 1,800 calories a day or more and not gaining bodyfat.

• You look leaner, with attractive muscular definition.

• Your appetite is so strong that you can't wait to eat all your calories.

• You can even "cheat" occasionally – and not regain bodyfat.

• Your energy level reaches an all-time high.

As you follow this program, be prepared for raised eyebrows and unrelenting criticism from your friends. "You can't possibly eat all that food," they'll say. "You're going to get so fat!"

Don't worry about responding to them. The results will speak for themselves.

Principle #2: Spread your calories throughout the day.

On this program, you eat five times a day – three full meals and two mini-meals of food or two "mock meals" consisting of a special protein/carbohydrate beverage. Don't be surprised or taken aback by this principle. Most people eat five or more times a day anyway, if you count coffee breaks and snacktime. The only difference here is that you'll be eating healthy, nutritious foods at each of your five meals. And, as you'll soon find out, each meal is a breeze to prepare.

Spreading your calories out over five meals is another important factor in changing your biochemistry to burn bodyfat. Consider the results of this research study, published in *The New England Journal of Medicine* (October 1989):

A group of men ate 2,700 calories a day over a three-week period, eating three meals daily. They took a two-week break and then returned. They again ate 2,700 calories a day but divided those calories into 17 small meals a day. They started losing bodyfat, and their metabolic rates increased significantly. Not only that, their levels of low density lipoproteins (LDL – also known as "bad cholesterol") dropped, and food absorption and utilization of nutrients were greatly enhanced.[10]

Did you know that every time you eat a meal your metabolic rate goes up? That's right, and the reason is that your system starts working very hard to turn that meal into fuel. As part of digestion and absorption, heat is given off in a process called thermogenesis, and this hikes your metabolism. So by eating frequent meals throughout the day, your metabolism is constantly charged up.

Principle #3: Choose metabolic-activating foods.

For your body to burn fat and produce energy, your metabolism has to be operating at peak levels. I call this a "metabolic roll." One of the key factors that starts a metabolic roll is calories – not only the amount you eat but also the kind of calories you eat.

Calories are derived from protein, carbohydrates, and fats. A diet too high in protein and too low in carbohydrates does not supply enough fuel for the body and results in a loss of lean body mass (muscle). Without enough carbohydrates to use for energy, your body draws on protein in the muscle for energy. Muscle tissue is lost as a result.

A diet high in carbohydrates and low in protein presents its own set of problems. Although you get an immediate lift from the high carbohydrate intake, your stamina drops fast in the absence of protein. As I explain in Chapter 5, protein combined with carbohydrates slows the digestion for a steady, even release of energy. Also, protein drives the metabolism. Without enough protein, your body is less able to burn fat.

In the Lean Bodies program, I classify the foods you eat into four groups: lean proteins, starchy carbohydrates, lean fibrous vegetables, and essential fatty acids (EFAs). These foods are explained in upcoming chapters. Each daily menu on the Lean Bodies program provides these foods in the following ratio:

Protein: 25%

Carbohydrates: 65%

Fat: 10%

Principle #4: Follow a program of moderate aerobic exercise.

One of the factors that has the most dramatic effect on metabolism is exercise. Many health professionals, however, promote the idea that it is perfectly acceptable to follow a low-calorie diet as long as you add exercise to speed up the metabolism. Nothing could be further from the truth! Exercise in the absence of adequate calories for fuel is actually detrimental to your health. Here is why:

Everyone needs a certain base number of calories each day just to exist, and this number is based on your Resting Metabolic Rate (RMR). (For more information on this, see Chapter 11.) Suppose you are a man who weighs 170 pounds. If you sit in a chair all day, you use 1,850 calories of energy to just breathe, to pump blood through your circulatory system, and to drive all the cellular processes that support life. By eating, you use up an additional 200 or more calories a day. Therefore, your daily caloric requirement – the base number of calories you need to just exist – is about 2,000 calories.

Let's carry this scenario a little further. Without increasing your caloric intake, you decide to start an aerobic exercise program, which uses up from 300 to 600 calories an hour, depending on how strenuous the exercise is. At this point, you're letting your body run on 1,400 to 1,700 calories a day – well below what you need to support your body's basic energy requirements or, in other words, to exist.

The point is: Inadequate calories combined with aerobic exercise suppresses your metabolism even more. I've worked with many women who tried to live on 800 calories a day, went to aerobic exercise classes every day, and then wondered why they couldn't lose bodyfat. Remember: Exercise will speed up your metabolism as long as you're eating enough calories to support your extra energy requirements.

Accompanied by adequate calories and proper nutrition, aerobic exercise has several beneficial results:

• It burns fat.

• It enhances your oxygen delivery system (oxygen is needed to burn fat).

• It increases muscle, a metabolically active body tissue.

• It improves the pumping action of your heart.

• It enlarges your major blood vessels so that more nutrients can be carried to body tissues and carbon dioxide can be transported away much faster.

Duration and timing of aerobic exercise maximize the effects of aerobics on your metabolism. An interesting study was recently conducted at the University of Victoria in British Columbia that underlines the important relationship between metabolism and the duration of aerobic exercise.

Five men rode a stationary bicycle at a moderate intensity, randomly varying the length of their rides each day in 30-minute, 45-minute, and 60-minute periods. The researchers found that after the 30-minute ride, the metabolism stayed elevated for 130 minutes; after the 45-minute ride, the metabolism stayed high for 205 minutes. Following the 60-minute ride, the metabolism remained elevated for 455 minutes – the equivalent of an extra 17 minutes of cycling.[11]

So to maximize fat burning, you should exercise aerobically several times a week for 45 to 60 minutes each session. Walking, running, riding a bicycle, exercising on a ski machine or stair-climber – these are all excellent choices. If you've never exercised, though, you'll need to gradually build up to 45 or 60 minutes of working out. Also, never begin an exercise program unless you've first consulted your physician.

Also important is the timing of your aerobic exercise. If you do aerobics for 45 to 60 minutes in the morning before your first meal, your body begins burning fatty acids (bodyfat) for energy because there is very little stored carbohydrate (glycogen) in the muscles to supply energy. You become leaner as a result. The carbohydrates you eat throughout the day are used to replenish the muscles with glycogen – and are not turned into bodyfat. Plus, the 45 to 60-minute aerobic session boosts your metabolism for the next seven hours. By following these duration/timing guidelines, along with frequent meals, you'll shed bodyfat much faster.

I also recommend that you consider weight training as an adjunct to your aerobic program. Weight training develops lean body mass (muscle), and the more lean mass you have, the faster your metabolism. More information on weight training and aerobic exercise is covered in Chapter 9.

Getting Lean

With the Lean Bodies program, you can successfully change the way you look and feel. Just think: No longer will you have to "starve" yourself to get in shape. You'll soon be free from the bonds of restrictive dieting. Before long, you'll know how to eat more of the right kind of calories and stay leaner and healthier than you have been in years.

❦ *Key Points*

- You can lose bodyfat – and keep it off – by increasing calories, not by cutting calories.

- Knowing your body composition (bodyfat to lean mass) is more important than knowing your weight as measured by the scales.

- Caloric restriction slows your metabolism, making it increasingly difficult to lose bodyfat.

- When you go on and off diets, your body starts producing more of an enzyme called lipoprotein lipase, or LPL, which steps up fat production and storage.

- Repetitive low-calorie dieting has serious health risks, including high blood pressure, heart disease, gallbladder disease, and a weakened immune response.

- Dangerous dieting practices such as vomiting and laxative abuse are addictive and health-damaging.

- You can change your biochemistry to burn bodyfat in four ways: (1) A gradual increase in calories. (2) Spreading calories throughout the day. (3) The selection of metabolic-activating foods. (4) A program of moderate exercise.

2

❦ Lean Protein: a Metabolic Activator

R I C K W. , a tennis coach, is one of the most active people I know. He is on the tennis courts about three hours every day, he coaches college-level tennis players, and he works out with weights and aerobic equipment six days a week. Despite his active lifestyle, Rick felt rundown about 90 percent of the time. He was so weak in the gym that he could barely do 25 push-ups. After an intense workout, he would reach a state of near collapse. At one point, he was even passing blood in his urine.

But like many active people, Rick believed he was eating nutritiously. His diet consisted of mostly fruits and vegetables, with about three ounces of protein every other day. "I was a near-vegetarian," he says.

Rick started the Lean Bodies program because he wanted more energy. Once on the program, he began to eat three to six ounces of protein three times a day, supplemented by a protein drink once a day.

The result was a gain of 10 pounds of solid muscle. At the same time, Rick reported that he felt stronger than ever before.

"Where once I couldn't even bench press 125 pounds, today I can lift 225 pounds," Rick says. "When I was 25 years old, I had trouble touching the rim of a basketball goal. I'm 40 now, and I can jump up and grab it. Those extra 10 pounds of muscle haven't slowed me down a bit. In fact, they've made me quicker. Once I started eating more protein, my body started performing more efficiently."

Prior to starting Lean Bodies, Rick was protein-deficient. Adding more protein to his diet resulted in a remarkable transformation. Of all nutrients, protein is the single most important one because it is found in every cell of your body. In fact, the word "protein" comes from a Greek word meaning "first." Unfortunately, though, protein has gotten a bad reputation over the years – a reputation it does not deserve. In 1991, for example, an advocacy group of physicians in Washington, D.C., declared that there should be a "New Four Food Groups," consisting of whole grains, vegetables, legumes, and fruit. Meat and dairy products, the group recommended, should be used only as seasonings and alternative foods, rather than as dietary staples.

This group claimed that high consumption of meats and other proteins shortens the life span, whereas a fruit/vegetable/whole grain-based diet increases longevity. Therefore, protein sources, they argued, should be dropped as a main food category.

Such a move can be described only as irresponsible. Protein is indispensable to life because it plays a role in every part of the body and in every cell. In fact, our bodies are constructed entirely of protein. The protein we eat is broken down into nitrogen-containing chemicals called amino acids. These are used to form muscle; hemoglobin, which carries oxygen to cells; enzymes and hormones, which regulate all body processes; and antibodies, which fight off infection and disease. At the cellular level, amino acids assist in the formation of chromosomes, which are bodies inside cells that carry DNA and RNA, the nucleo-proteins that control cellular growth and reproduction, thus governing all life.

The argument that high protein diets are linked to shortened life just does not hold up. Take the Eskimos, for example. They eat enormous amounts of protein, namely ocean-going white fish, and in much higher quantities than other Americans consume. Yet life-threatening diseases such as coronary thrombosis are unheard-of in Eskimo populations.

It is important to emphasize that the real culprit in heart disease and other food-related illnesses is not protein. It is saturated fat, which leads to a dangerous build-up of cholesterol in the arteries.

Some researchers, however, point to the low cholesterol counts found in Oriental populations as proof of the benefits of a low-protein diet. But because the Oriental-type diet consists primarily of vegetables and grains, it is very low in fat – and that is the reason for these low cholesterol counts.

Still, an Oriental diet is not the answer, and the proof is in the performance of Chinese athletes. It is a well-known fact in sports circles that Chinese athletes have very little stamina. They get out of the gate fast but soon falter due to poor endurance. Research is now showing that athletes need much more protein than non-athletes for endurance and energy. Oriental diets do not supply enough protein to support the energy systems of the body.

Interestingly, life-threatening illnesses such as cardiovascular disease, hypertension, and diabetes were virtually unknown among early man. It has been estimated that these people consumed 3,000 calories a day, with a diet that consisted of 35 percent meat (more than twice the consumption of the average American) and 65 percent vegetables. Their fat intake was quite low because they ate game animals, which provide very lean sources of protein.[1]

Five Vital Reasons Why You Need Protein

Low protein diets can have many adverse effects on health. So that you can understand why, here is a closer look at what protein does in the body.

(1) *Protein is essential for growth and maintenance.*

Your body is in a perpetual state of growth and repair. When you wash your face, whole cells are sloughed off from the surface of your skin. After you cut your hair or fingernails, new growth occurs. Similarly, other cells of the body, which die or are lost through normal physiological processes, must constantly be replaced. Protein is required to build new cells to replace those that are lost.

Because your body is constructed of protein, you must have protein from food to "reconstruct" it because amino acids in food are the only available source of protein.

In addition, protein provides the foundation for the construction of bones, teeth, and scar tissue. For these tissues to form, a protein matrix called collagen, which creates cartilage, must first be set down. Crystals of minerals such as calcium, phosphorus, and fluoride are deposited in this matrix, and hardened bones and teeth begin to form. Collagen is also the mending protein that forms scars to bond separated tissues. Ligaments and tendons are composed of the protein collagen. Additionally, it is a strengthening component between the cells of vein and artery walls.

(2) *Protein drives your body's catabolism / anabolism cycle.*

When you exercise, your muscle tissue is broken down in a process called catabolism and later rebuilt in a process called anabolism. Protein drives these processes, known as the catabolism / anabolism cycle.

When protein intake is increased, your body actually starts to form new lean muscle. This occurs in the anabolic portion of the cycle.

Prior to starting the program, one of my clients had always race-walked for 45 minutes each day while following a low-calorie diet. Despite this rigorous exercise program, her muscles still lacked tone. She was not taking in enough protein to rebuild muscle after the catabolic breakdown caused by exercise. Her muscles were in a perpetual state of catabolism.

After three weeks on the program, she flexed her legs for us. Her quadriceps and calves were lean and hard, all because she was getting enough protein to build lean tissue. Every ounce of lean tissue you put on as a result of catabolism/anabolism is an insurance policy against bodyfat coming back on.

Day after day, this cycle repeats itself, and as long as there is sufficient protein to repair and rebuild, the building of muscle tissue continues.

(3) *Protein has a high "specific dynamic action" on the metabolism.*

After you eat a meal, your metabolic rate increases – a reaction partly due to the various chemical reactions associated with digestion, absorption, and storage of food in the body. Another reason for the increase is that certain amino acids in food directly stimulate cellular processes.

A high carbohydrate meal boosts your metabolic rate about 4 percent, while a high protein meal raises the metabolism about 30 percent above normal, usually within one hour after the meal. This can last for as long as three to 12 hours. This effect of protein on metabolic rate is called "specific dynamic action."[2]

(4) *Protein helps regulate your body's water balance.*

If it were possible to travel by boat through your body tissues, you would find water in three areas: between the cells, within the cells, and inside your capillaries, veins, and arteries (the vascular system). In healthy people, protein, working together with certain minerals, helps regulate the proper amount of water in each area. This happens because proteins are "hydrophilic," or attracted to water. Water molecules thus tend to congregate near the proteins.

When your diet is protein-deficient, proteins in the blood become depleted. Without enough protein to cling to, water in the vascular spaces leaks out into the spaces between the cells. Once there, it cannot be excreted by the kidneys, and the result is edema or water retention.

The way to prevent this is to have adequate amounts of protein in your diet and to drink plenty of water (eight to 10 large glasses a day). The more water you drink, the more you make available to your vascular system. This system circulates water through your kidneys, where it can be properly excreted.

(5) *Protein strengthens the immune system.*

Dietary proteins produce other proteins called antibodies, which are found in the blood and which combat disease. When your body is attacked by viruses, bacteria, or other foreign agents, antibodies inactivate the invader, thus warding off the disease. Once your body has produced antibodies against an invading agent, your cells keep a molecular memory of how to fight it the next time that infection sets in.

In addition to producing antibodies, protein strengthens immunity in many other ways. Many studies have been done on protein status and immune function. The findings show that inadequate protein:

• Interferes with the function of lymphocytes, a type of white blood cell formed in the lymphatic system. Lymphocytes are responsible for promoting immunity at the cellular level.

• Impedes the action of macrophages. These are cells involved in the production of antibodies, which help the body combat foreign invaders that cause disease. Macrophages also play a key role in cellular immunity.

• Decreases the function of leukocytes, another type of white blood cell, causing slower cellular metabolism and weakened resistance to bacterial invasion.

• Increases tumor formation.

These findings speak for themselves: Clearly, building immunity against disease requires an ample supply of dietary protein.

Complete Protein for Excellent Health

The amino acids found in protein are of two types: indispensable amino acids and dispensable amino acids. You get indispensable amino acids from animal sources – meat, poultry, fish, milk and milk products, and eggs – in the right proportions in which your body needs them. And your body is capable of synthesizing dispensable amino acids on its own.

Plant sources of protein such as rice, potatoes, and legumes are low in one or more indispensable amino acids and by themselves do not provide a good balance. You would have to eat a pound of potatoes, for example, to equal the amino acid content found in one ounce of chicken.

The following chart lists these amino acids, along with their specific functions.

Indispensable Amino Acids

Methionine. Involved in the synthesis of choline (a B-complex vitamin), which helps prevent the build-up of fat in the liver.

Lysine. Involved in protein synthesis, including muscle and collagen formation.

Arginine. Stimulates the release of growth hormone in the body. Necessary for growth in children.

Threonine. Involved in energy production.

Tryptophan. Produces a number of physiologically important substances in the body. Converted to serotonin in the body, a neurotransmitter that relays nerve impulses.

Isoleucine. A branched chain amino acid that assists the muscles in synthesizing other amino acids.

Leucine. A branched chain amino acid that assists the muscles in synthesizing other amino acids.

Histidine. Involved in protein synthesis. Necessary for growth in children.

Valine. A branched chain amino acid that assists the muscles in synthesizing other amino acids.

Phenylalanine. Helps produce and activate pain-suppressing hormones called endorphins.

Dispensable Amino Acids

Glycine. Helps synthesize other dispensable amino acids for use by the body and is an important constituent of red blood cells.

Alanine. Involved in the production of energy and stabilization of blood sugar levels.

Serine. Involved in cellular energy production and is required for the function of certain neurotransmitters.

Cysteine. Involved in protein synthesis. Protects the body from oxidative damage.

Aspartic acid. Helps extend energy by reducing levels of ammonia (a by-product of intense exercise) in the blood.

Glutamic acid. Involved in energy production, helps transport potassium to the brain and works together with other nutrients such as B-complex vitamins and magnesium.

Cystine. Involved in the action of antioxidants.

Tyrosine. Used to manufacture adrenaline and thyroid hormones.

Proline. Used to construct collagen.

Hydroxyproline. A constituent of proteins such as collagen.

Many amino acids depend on vitamins and minerals to do their jobs. One example is the amino acid methionine, which assists in the removal of toxins from the liver and in the regeneration of liver and kidney tissue. It relies on vitamin B_6 and magnesium for its action. Lysine works together with vitamin C to manufacture L-carnitine, which enables muscle cells to use oxygen more efficiently.

Your body continually takes apart amino acids in foods and then uses them to create new protein – in your blood, in your hair and fingernails, and in your muscles. In fact, your body cannot manufacture protein unless all of the indispensable amino acids are present.

Foods are graded for protein quality in two ways: (1) their digestibility and absorbability, and (2) the number of indispensable amino acids present. Egg protein, for example, has a grade of 100 and, as the "perfect protein," is what all other proteins are judged against. Any protein with a grade of 70 or above is considered a high quality protein. Chicken and fish, for example, have scores of 75.

The lean protein you eat on this program is high quality protein, derived from animal sources, and referred to as "complete protein" (that is, it supplies all the indispensable amino acids you need for excellent health). High quality protein is well utilized by the body. For example, between 90 and 95 percent of the protein from animal sources is absorbed by the body, whereas only 73 percent of the protein in plant sources is absorbed.

Lean Bodies Protein

Twenty-five percent (25%) of your daily food intake on the Lean

Bodies program comes from protein sources. According to new research, people who are more active may require slightly more protein, as much as 30 percent. Your protein choices on the Lean Bodies program are:

Egg whites. The whites are the leanest and healthiest portion of the egg. A surprising fact is that every time you eat a whole egg, your cholesterol goes up 10 percent.[3] Most of that cholesterol is concentrated in the egg yolk. That is why you eat only the egg whites on this program.

White meat poultry (skinless chicken and turkey). This protein source is very high in several of the B-complex vitamins, iron, phosphorus, and zinc. Also, eating skinless chicken (as well as fish), instead of fatty meats, appears to lower your risk of colon cancer. That is the finding of a study that monitored the diet and health of 88,751 women over six years. The highest risk of colon cancer was linked with high consumption of beef, pork, and lamb.[4]

The best ways to prepare white meat chicken and turkey are baking, broiling, grilling, or microwaving.

Fish. This is one of the leanest sources of protein around. Besides being low in fat, fish is the most abundant source of omega-3 fatty acids, which help prevent blood clots and plaque buildup on arterial walls – contributing factors to heart disease and stroke. Omega-3 fatty acids also appear to increase white cell activity, thus boosting the body's defense against disease. All fish provides a certain amount of omega-3 fatty acids, but cold-water fish such as halibut, salmon, and rainbow trout tends to be higher. Fish is also a rich source of vitamins and minerals, including vitamin B_{12}, calcium, phosphorus, zinc, and selenium.

The best ways to prepare fish are broiling, baking, poaching, steaming, and grilling. For some delicious fish recipes, see Appendix

B, Lean Bodies Cooking. Your fish choices on the Lean Bodies program are:

Bass

Catfish

Cod

Flounder

Grouper

Halibut

Haddock

Hake

Mackerel

Mahi Mahi

Marlin

Ocean Perch

Orange Roughy

Red Snapper

Salmon

Scrod (Boston)

Shark

Shrimp

Sole

Swordfish

Trout

Tuna

What About Red Meat?

Although an excellent source of iron, vitamin B_{12}, and protein, red meats are riddled with saturated fat, making them a poor choice if you are trying to lose bodyfat. Unless your physician has diagnosed you as an anemic (low iron in the blood), eliminate these. Lean cuts such as eye-of-the-round, tenderloin, and filet mignon may be re-introduced after the first seven weeks of the program.

Water, Water, and More Water

Because your daily protein intake is high on this program, you must drink eight to 10 large glasses of water every day. Like all foods, protein generates metabolic waste products that must be dissolved in water and removed by the kidneys. Without enough water, the kidneys cannot efficiently remove those wastes, and damage to the kidneys may occur. It is important to point out too that high protein intake is not harmful to the kidneys — as long as you are healthy.[5] In fact, anyone with healthy kidneys can handle more protein as long as plenty of water is taken in.

In addition to waste removal, water has many other vital functions in the body. It serves as a medium for every enzymatic and chemical reaction in the body, including the digestion of food and the metabolism of fat, and it transports nutrients and oxygen to every cell in the body.

More than 75 percent of your body is made up of water. You can survive without food for days, but, without water, dehydration begins in just a few hours. Next to oxygen, water is the substance most important for life. The best source of water is natural spring water. I do not recommend distilled water, even though it is purified, because all the minerals are removed from it during the vaporization and condensation process.

Coffee is not a good source of water either because it contains caffeine, which adversely affects the brain and the nervous system. Physiologically, caffeine triggers the release of stimulating chemicals from the adrenal glands into the bloodstream, elevating blood sugar. In turn, this causes blood vessels to constrict and the blood pressure to go up by as much as ten percent. Coffee also increases the output of stomach acid, which makes urine more acidic, and increases the excretion of magnesium, a vital mineral. A magnesium deficiency can cause nervousness, tight muscles, bone loss, and cardiac arrhythmias. There is also some evidence that coffee can inhibit the absorption of iron and the B-complex vitamin thiamine.

If you are accustomed to drinking coffee, I suggest that you gradually wean yourself from it. Once you start feeling more energetic on this program, your need for coffee should disappear.

❘ *Key Points*

- Protein is the single most important nutrient because it is a constituent of every cell in your body.

- Saturated fat, not protein, is the culprit in heart disease and other illnesses related to diet.

- There are five vital reasons why you need protein: for growth and maintenance, to drive the catabolism/anabolism cycle, to activate your metabolism, to regulate water balance, and to strengthen your immune system.

- The protein on the Lean Bodies program is complete, supplying all the indispensable amino acids needed for excellent health.

- Your lean proteins on the program are egg whites, white meat chicken and turkey, and fish and shrimp.

- Drink eight to 10 glasses of water a day.

- On the Lean Bodies program, approximately 25 percent of your daily food intake comes from lean proteins.

3

¶ *Carbohydrates: Fuel and Fiber*

MEDICAL PROBLEMS associated with the birth of her second child left Cindy W. with lingering fatigue. "By 10 o'clock in the morning, I looked like all the blood had drained from my body," she remembers. "Every morning I woke up in disbelief that I had lived through the night. That's how tired and sick I was."

Cindy consulted with me about her problem, and I suggested a nutritional program for her, which included eating more nutrient-rich foods and avoiding processed foods. She took my advice, and soon her energy and endurance returned. A few years later, however, she decided to cut her calories to 500 a day to lose weight quickly. As a result, her fatigue returned.

Cindy decided to start the Lean Bodies program with the hope of regaining her energy. In just a few weeks, she did. In fact, she felt so energized that she decided to take up running. Now she runs in marathons.

You may not want to be a marathon runner like Cindy, but if you are like most people, you want to feel energetic throughout the day. That is where carbohydrates fit in.

Carbohydrates are energy foods. During digestion, they are changed into glucose (blood sugar), which circulates in the blood and is used as energy for the red blood cells and the central nervous system. Glucose not used right away is stored in the liver and muscles as glycogen. When your muscles do not have enough glycogen, you feel tired and fatigued.

Carbohydrates are divided into two groups: simple sugars — found in candies, syrups, fruits and fruit juices, and processed foods — and complex carbohydrates — found in whole grains, beans, and vegetables. Simple sugars and complex carbohydrates yield the same amount of food energy, but that is where the similarity ends. In fact, it is a common misconception that once a carbohydrate — any type of carbohydrate — is broken down into glucose, the body does not differentiate the source of that carbohydrate and uses it in the same way. Not true. Simple sugars and complex carbohydrates are not handled equally by the body, due to the differences in their molecular structure.

Simple sugars, for example, are constructed of either single (monosaccharide) or double (disaccharide) molecules of sugar. Complex carbohydrates are polysaccharides, meaning that they contain a large number of sugar molecules linked together in long chains. These differences in structure play a major role in how carbohydrates are absorbed and utilized. Certain carbohydrates, for instance, are more readily converted to bodyfat. Naturally, those are the ones you want to avoid. Here is a closer look.

Simple Sugars

Six types of simple sugars are found in foods, and the monosaccharide glucose is one of these. Another monosaccharide is fructose, which gives fruits and fruit juices their sweet taste. Galactose, also a monosaccharide, is seldom found by itself in nature but is instead a part of lactose, a simple sugar in milk.

The other three sugars are disaccharides, which are pairs of monosaccharides bonded together. The most common disaccharide is sucrose or table sugar. At the molecular level, sucrose is composed of glucose and fructose, making it the sweetest of all sugars. Found in sugar cane and sugar beets, sucrose is purified and refined to provide the various sugar products you see on the grocery store shelves. Sucrose is a principal ingredient in candy, cakes, cookies, and other sweets.

Lactose, which is made up of glucose and galactose, is the principal sugar found in milk. You may be familiar with the term "lactose-intolerant." This is an inherited or acquired condition in which individuals cannot digest lactose. They fail to produce the enzyme lactase, which is required for the breakdown of lactose in the body.

Maltose or malt sugar is the third type of disaccharide, and it is constructed from two units of glucose. Maltose is found in plants during the early stages of germination.

The Conversion Factor

Certain foods are easily converted into bodyfat by your body, and simple sugars are one of these foods. Simple sugars are rapidly released into the system, driving your blood sugar up too high and giving you a quick "rush" followed by a fast "crash." The first organ to react to this sugar overload is the pancreas, which responds by secreting more of the hormone insulin into the bloodstream. Insulin activates fat cell enzymes, facilitating the movement of fat from the bloodstream into fat cells for storage. Additionally, insulin prevents glucagon (a hormone that opposes the action of insulin) from entering the bloodstream, and glucagon is responsible for unlocking fat stores. The cumulative result of these interactions is the ready conversion of simple sugars to bodyfat. (Another food that converts easily to bodyfat is dietary fat. When you eat simple sugars and fat at the same meal, fat storage is speeded up.)

A little known fact is that certain fruits and fruit juices can be culprits in promoting bodyfat – even though they are highly nutritious, full of vitamins, minerals, and fiber. As mentioned, however, these foods are simple sugars because they contain fructose.

Molecularly, fructose is put together differently from glucose and, consequently, your body uses it differently. After being absorbed into the bloodstream, fructose goes directly to the liver where it is metabolized into triglycerides, a fat. In fact, research has shown that fructose elevates triglyceride levels in the blood in susceptible individuals.[1]

Before going on the Lean Bodies program, Kathy S. was a confirmed sweets lover, even though she had already given up both white flour and white sugar. To satisfy her sweet tooth, she started eating fruit juice-sweetened foods available at the health store where she worked. "I could justify eating those because I thought they were healthy," she says. But gradually, her weight started climbing, and I suspect it was because of all the "healthy sweets" she was eating.

Kathy started the program, gradually upping her calories to 2500 a day and using the nutritional supplements I recommend. Before long, friends were noticing that Kathy had lost weight – and complimenting her on it. But in reality, she had gained 10 pounds of lean mass! "I was at 19-percent bodyfat, and I looked better than I did in high school," she says.

This all goes to show the effect that too much fruit can have on the metabolism – and what the right foods can do for you. For peak metabolic efficiency, you should avoid simple sugars, including most fruits and fruit juices, during the first seven weeks of the Lean Bodies program. From a concentrated sugar standpoint, there is no difference between drinking a glass of orange juice and a can of cola. Both are simple sugars that produce the quick rush/fast crash reaction – and thus the production of insulin and the corresponding suppression of glucagon.

During the first seven weeks on the Lean Bodies program, eat the following fruits: Granny Smith apples, green apples, strawberries, blackberries, blueberries, cranberries, boysenberries, or pears. Be sure to eat them with the peel, which is high in fiber. These fruits contain fewer simple carbohydrates (and consequently are less sweet), more fiber, and more water than fruits such as bananas, grapes, raisins, and oranges. Our experience shows that when people in our Lean Bodies classes choose the less sweet fruits over other fruits during the first seven weeks of the program, they lose body fat faster. Later, when your metabolism is faster and your calories are being processed more efficiently, you can add the sweeter fruits back into your diet.

Dairy products are another group of foods that are restricted on the Lean Bodies program during the first seven weeks. I recommend that you eat up to eight ounces a day of non-fat milk, skim milk, and plain, non-fat yogurt (unless you have lactose-intolerance). These are good sources of calcium, which is also supplied by vegetables such as kale, turnip greens, collard greens, broccoli, and other green, leafy vegetables.

Remember, dairy products contain the milk sugar lactose, which, like all simple sugars, is readily converted to bodyfat. Other dairy products such as cheese, whole milk, and cream are high in fat, which is easily converted to bodyfat.

Please note: Pregnant and lactating women and growing children should not exclude dairy products from their diets.

To sum up, simple sugars easily convert to bodyfat and must be avoided. Complex carbohydrates, on the other hand, do not easily turn into bodyfat. There are two types of complex carbohydrates you eat on the Lean Bodies program: starchy carbohydrates and lean, fibrous vegetables. Together, these carbohydrates supply 65 percent of your total food intake.

Starchy Carbohydrates

Starchy carbohydrates are natural, unrefined whole grains such as brown rice and oatmeal; beans and legumes such as kidney beans, lentils, and peas; and tubers such as potatoes and yams. As polysaccharides, starchy carbohydrates are chains of dozens of glucose molecules linked together. Because of this complex molecular structure, more energy is required for starchy carbohydrates to be digested, absorbed, and utilized by the body. The glucose from starchy carbohydrates, therefore, enters the system much more slowly than glucose from simple sugars, allows minimal production of insulin, and provides more sustained energy levels.

Even among starchy carbohydrates, there are different rates of release. Potatoes, for example, release glucose faster than yams, lentils, and some beans. But because on the Lean Bodies program starchy carbohydrates are always eaten with lean protein sources (a slowly digested food), the rate of glucose release is delayed even more, and your energy levels are more steady as a result. This special way of combining your foods is explained in Chapter 5.

Your starchy carbohydrate choices on this program are:

Barley

Brown rice

Buckwheat

Bulghur (cracked wheat)

Butter beans

Chard

Chick peas

Corn

Garbanzo beans

Kasha

Kidney beans

Legumes

Lentils

Lima beans

Millet

Old-fashioned rolled oats

Peas

Pinto beans

Potatoes

Rice cakes

Sweet potatoes

White beans

*Winter squash

Yams

Any natural, unrefined whole grain

The Problem with Processed Carbohydrates

Breads, pasta, and bagels are initially excluded from the Lean Bodies program. Even though many of these foods are nutritious, they are more "processed," which means they are easily converted to sugar and then to bodyfat. In addition, processed foods do not have as high a nutrient level as natural, unrefined foods. During the first seven weeks of this program, stay away from bread, pasta, and bagels. Once you are eating 1,800 calories a day or more, you will not miss these foods. Later on, however, you will be able to reintroduce bread into

---

Although winter squash is classified here as a starchy carbohydrate, it is very high in fiber – so I also count it as a lean, fibrous vegetable.

your diet. This bread should be of the whole-grain variety because it
is rich in nutrients and fiber.

Lean, Fibrous Vegetables

Lean, fibrous vegetables are the second important type of carbohydrate on my program. Low in calories, these vegetables supply
minerals and fiber. Minerals help form body structures such as bones,
teeth, and tissues and are involved in all the body's metabolic processes. Fiber is needed to maintain the health of your digestive system
– in addition to performing a number of other important functions.

Several of the lean, fibrous vegetables on the Lean Bodies program fall into the category of "cruciferous vegetables," and these
include broccoli, broccoflower (a hybrid of broccoli and cauliflower),
cabbage, bok choy, cauliflower, brussels sprouts, and watercress.

Cruciferous vegetables are rich in vitamin A, calcium, and fiber –
nutrients which appear to have cancer-protective effects. Studies have
shown that eating these vegetables lowers the risk of stomach, breast,
and intestinal cancers. [2]

You may eat a wide variety of lean, fibrous vegetables on this
program, including:

Alfalfa Sprouts
Artichokes
Asparagus
Bamboo shoots
Bok choy (Chinese cabbage)
Broccoli
Broccoflower
Brussels sprouts
Cabbage
Cauliflower

Carrots

Collard greens

Eggplant

Green beans

Green, leafy vegetables (with the exception of iceberg lettuce, which has less nutritional value)

Kale

Leeks

Mushrooms

Okra

Onions

Parsley

Parsnips

Rutabaga

Salad vegetables

Scallions

Spinach

Summer squash

Turnips

Turnip greens

Watercress

Zucchini

The Fiber Link

In ancient times, people ground their own grain using two flat stones, and the result was a coarse yet digestible food. In 450 B.C., the Greeks developed millstones, powered by water. Later, the Romans improved on this technology by adding gears to the apparatus, allowing them to run several millstones at a time. Later, windmills became the chief method of milling grain.

The flour obtained from all of these early technologies was highly nutritious because of its coarseness. Yet it spoiled quickly, and millers began to seek ways to solve this spoilage problem. In the 1840s, with the advent of the Industrial Revolution, giant steel rollers replaced the primitive millstone. The new technology allowed modern millers to extract the wheat's germ, the most nutritious part of the seed. The by-product of this new germless flour did not spoil as quickly.

Next came air sifters, which further purified the flour by removing the bran from the wheat. What was left was pure white flour as we know it today. Tons of this new white flour was imported to every corner of the world, and less than five percent of the population continued to eat the dark, coarser bread, once popular in Europe.

Not long after the worldwide introduction of white flour, a disease called beri beri began to appear, particularly among the poor. The disease is a deficiency of thiamine, a B-complex vitamin supplied by whole grains.

In 1906, scientists discovered that our foods contain certain substances, which they called "vitamins," that are necessary for our health. Deficiency diseases such as beri beri were linked with the low nutrient content of white flour. To remedy the problem, four synthetic nutrients were put into the flour: iron, riboflavin, niacin, and thiamine. This replacement was intended to "enrich" our white flour products.

Deficiency diseases continued, nonetheless. In 1910, appendectomy was the most common surgery of the day. Interestingly, Dr. Charles Mayo informed the 1924 National Conference of the American Medical Association that appendicitis was rare in past ages yet had become a disease of modern man.

As our foods became even more processed, they became devitalized. Grains, in particular, lost most of their fiber – a loss contributing to deadly digestive tract illnesses. By 1950, for example, colon cancer had become the second leading cancer-causing death – and still is today, according to the National Cancer Institute.[3]

Fiber is a nutrient necessary for good health. It absorbs moisture in the body and adds bulk to the feces. In the absence of fiber, food moves slowly through the system, putrefying in the body and eventually creating stools that are difficult to pass. A high fiber diet, on the other hand, keeps the digestive system healthy and may even enhance fat loss. A study of the African Bantu tribe showed that the natives ate an average of 3,000 calories a day (well above the average consumption of our population) yet there was no obesity. The researchers concluded that this phenomenon was the result of the Bantu's high fiber diet and high level of activity.[4]

Starchy carbohydrates and lean, fibrous vegetables are excellent sources of fiber. There are two types of fibers in these foods, each with different health effects: water-soluble fiber and water-insoluble fiber. Water-soluble fibers include gums, a gelatinous polysaccharide in plants; pectins, a substance that binds cell walls in plant tissues; mucilages, a protein/polysaccharide; and hemicelluloses, a polysaccharide. These have been shown to reduce cholesterol levels and to slow the release of glucose into the bloodstream following a meal. Good sources of water-soluble fiber include rice, oatmeal, barley, corn, legumes, and carrots.[5]

Water-insoluble fibers include lignins, a constituent of plant cells that holds them together; cellulose, a polysaccharide found in the cell walls of plants; and some hemicelluloses. These fibers supply the bulk that keeps foods moving through the digestive system more quickly. Good sources of water-insoluble fiber include leafy vegetables, root vegetables, whole grains, and legumes.[6]

From a health standpoint, it is generally recommended that you eat between 20 to 35 grams a day of fiber from both water-soluble and water-insoluble sources. The Lean Bodies program provides this quantity of fiber.

❦ *Key Points*

• Carbohydrates are energy foods, which are converted into glucose for use by red blood cells, the central nervous system, the muscles, and the liver.

• There are two broad classifications of carbohydrates: simple sugars and complex carbohydrates, each used differently by your body. Simple sugars can convert readily to bodyfat because of their molecular structure and fast release into the body. Because it takes more energy to digest, absorb, and utilize complex carbohydrates, they are less likely to turn into bodyfat.

• Fruit and fruit juices contain the simple sugar fructose, which is metabolized into fat by the liver. To maximize fat-burning, limit your fruit intake to an occasional green apple or serving of berries during the first seven weeks of the Lean Bodies program. These contain less fructose than other fruits.

• The Lean Bodies program features two types of complex carbohydrates: starchy carbohydrates and lean, fibrous vegetables. These are rich in nutrients, including vitamins, minerals, and fiber (both water- soluble fiber and water-insoluble fiber).

• Processed carbohydrates such as breads and pastas should be avoided initially because they convert easily to sugar and then to bodyfat.

• On the Lean Bodies program, 65 percent of your daily food intake comes from starchy carbohydrates and lean, fibrous vegetables.

4

❡ EFAs and MCTs: the Healthy Fats

YOU HAVE PROBABLY BEEN TOLD that dietary fats are the "bad guys" when it comes to nutrition. Not all fats are bad, however. Certain fats are vital to health. The fats I am referring to are essential fatty acids or EFAs, which are made up of compounds called oleic acid, linoleic acid, linolenic acid, and arachidonic acid, all contained primarily in vegetable oils. Omega-3 fatty acids are another type of EFA, and they are found in fish.

All EFAs are vitamin-like substances that have a protective effect on the body. The reason these fats are called "essential" is because your body cannot manufacture them; you must obtain them from the foods you eat. EFAs are the "good guys" in the nutrition story. To understand why EFAs are beneficial, as well as why other fats are harmful, it helps to look at the structure of fats and their utilization by the body.

The Chemical Composition of Fats

Fats are constructed of fatty acids, which are made up of chains of carbon atoms with hydrogen atoms attached and with an acid group at one end. Think of this configuration as a charm bracelet. The carbons form the chain, and the hydrogen and the acid group are the charms.

The lengths of these chains vary according to the fat. Fats found in meat, for example, usually have chains that are 16 or more carbons long. Some carbon chains are much shorter, with six, eight, 10, or 12 carbon atoms.

When a fatty acid carries the maximum number of hydrogen atoms, it is loaded or "saturated." You can tell if a fat is saturated because it is solid at room temperature. Saturated fats are found in meats, dairy products, and lard. Your body can manufacture saturated fats, but the extra you take in can lead to coronary heart disease.

Other fatty acids are "unsaturated," and there are two types – monounsaturated and polyunsaturated. Monounsaturated fatty acids lack two hydrogen atoms. This type of fat is found in such foods as olive oil, olives, avocados, cashew nuts, and cold-water fish such as salmon, mackerel, halibut, and swordfish. Polyunsaturated fatty acids lack four or more hydrogen atoms and are found in fish and in most vegetable oils.

Unsaturated fats contain essential fatty acids (EFAs). They have very specific roles to play in maintaining health. For example:

Cellular health. EFAs protect the integrity of cell walls, making them flexible enough so that important materials such as nutrients and hormones can be exchanged from inside and outside the cell. Without adequate EFAs, cell walls become too rigid, and materials cannot easily pass in and out.

Fat mobilization. EFAs help mobilize cholesterol (a type of fat) and other fats from the body. Even though not an EFA, cholesterol is needed for health. It is involved in the synthesis of vitamin D for use by the body; it helps make myelin, the coating around nerves; it synthesizes bile, a substance involved in the digestion and absorption of fats; and it helps manufacture hormones.

In the body, cholesterol molecules attach to EFAs and are ferried through the bloodstream. As a result of this linkage, cholesterol can be changed into bile salts, which are required in the digestion of fats. Unless this happens, the body cannot properly dispose of cholesterol.

When EFAs are unavailable, the cholesterol molecules latch onto saturated fat molecules and can end up as plaque on the inner wall of the arteries.

Prostaglandins. EFAs are needed to produce prostaglandins. These are hormone-like substances that regulate nearly every system in your body, including your cardiovascular, immune, endocrine, central nervous, digestive, and reproductive systems. When EFAs are in ample supply, your entire body functions much better. In addition, immunity to disease and infection is greatly increased.

EFA Deficiencies

Signs of an EFA deficiency are dry, flaky skin and stiff, painful joints. These symptoms may indicate that your heart, brain, liver, and internal organs are EFA-deficient as well.

One woman in my program lost a substantial amount of bodyfat. Though delighted with the fat loss, she was concerned over the dryness of her skin and hair. When asked about her EFA intake, she admitted to not taking her safflower oil (one of the permissible EFAs on this program). I encouraged her to start using it in her diet, and just one week later, she reported marked improvement in her skin and hair.

Another case involved a competitive female bodybuilder, who complained that her hair was falling out, her skin had become extremely dry, and her joints were stiff. After observing her physical characteristics, I suspected that she was suffering from an EFA deficiency. This deficiency was aggravated by a restrictive diet in which she kept her calories and fats too low.

I put her on one tablespoon of flaxseed oil and six capsules of Evening Primrose Oil a day (a natural source of gamma-linolenic acid and linoleic acid). Two weeks later, her hair stopped falling out and her skin was smooth and glowing. Not only that, her joint stiffness disappeared all together. EFAs have also been shown to alleviate symptoms of premenstrual tension (PMS). Examples of physical symptoms include fluid retention; weight gain; swollen ankles, legs, and fingers; painful breasts; headaches and backaches; skin problems; and food cravings. Mental symptoms of PMS are depression, tension, irritability, lethargy, weeping, tantrums, and lack of concentration.

In 1981, a study was conducted at a major PMS clinic in Great Britain where 65 PMS sufferers were treated with Evening Primrose Oil. The starting dose was two capsules twice a day taken with food. More severe cases were treated with three capsules a day. Vitamin B_6 was administered at the same time. Treatment began three days before the symptoms typically appeared.

The results were encouraging: 61 percent of the women experienced complete relief of their symptoms; 23 percent, partial relief; and 15 percent, no change. One symptom in particular – breast discomfort – was improved in 72 percent of the cases. Other symptoms showing improvement were mood swings, anxiety, irritability, headaches, and fluid retention.

The women in this study were possibly deficient in EFAs, or their individual biochemistry required more EFAs than the general population. These deficiencies can lead to an apparent excess in the production of prolactin, a female hormone that is responsible for changes in mood and fluid metabolism. EFAs counteract the effects of prolactin.[1]

How Much Fat?

On the Lean Bodies program, 10 percent of your total food intake comes from dietary fats. One of the main reasons for this low ratio is that dietary fat, which like simple sugars, is easily converted to bodyfat. In fact, your body uses up less energy (3 percent) storing fat calories as bodyfat than it does storing calories from carbohydrates (25 percent).

Each day, add one teaspoon of an EFA source to your diet. This will guard against an EFA deficiency. The best sources are:

Flaxseed oil

Safflower oil

Canola oil

Linseed oil

Hain All-Blend

Evening Primrose oil (four to six capsules daily)

MCT Oil – the "Fatless Fat"

It is a well-known fact that dietary fat enhances the flavor of food. That is one of the reasons why Americans have such a big appetite for fatty food – and why limiting fat is so difficult for many people. Unfortunately, excess dietary fat turns into excess bodyfat. But what if there were a fat that did not easily get converted into bodyfat? There is, and it is called MCT oil, which stands for "medium chain triglyceride."

Available in fitness or sports nutrition centers, MCT oil is a 100 percent natural product refined from coconut oil through a special distillation process. It does not, however, have any of the adverse properties associated with tropical oils. MCT oil occurs naturally in many of the foods we eat and happens to be quite plentiful in human milk. The MCT oil used on the Lean Bodies program is an excellent product called CapTri® manufactured by Parrillo Performance of Cincinnati, Ohio. It tastes delicious when used as a salad dressing or poured on vegetables. You can even cook with it. (Ordering information is provided in Appendix C.)

MCT oil was first introduced more than 30 years ago in hospital feeding programs for patients and infants who had trouble digesting regular fats. Today, MCT oil has captured the attention of researchers who are interested in its use as a dietary supplement.

At 114 calories a tablespoon, MCT oil is a good source of extra calories when you are trying to gradually increase your caloric intake. But unlike conventional fats, calories from MCT oil are not easily stored as bodyfat.[2] This is why MCT oil is often referred to as the "fatless fat." To understand why, it helps to draw some comparisons between MCT oil and conventional fats such as butter, margarine, and vegetable oil. As I have explained, conventional fats are constructed of long carbon chains, with 16 or more carbon atoms strung together. Because of this structure, such fats are known as "long chain triglycerides" (LCTs). Bodyfat is also an LCT. MCT oil, on the other hand, has a much shorter carbon chain of only six to 12 carbon atoms, thus the name "medium chain triglycerides" or MCTs. These molecular differences cause MCTs and LCTs to be used quite differently by the body.

To be digested, LCTs must first be broken down in the watery medium of the intestines. This is an elaborate process because LCTs, like most oils, do not dissolve in water by themselves. They require bile salts, which are secreted by the gallbladder. In a process called emulsification, a molecule of bile acid attaches itself to a molecule of fat, dispersing the fat into the watery solution where it can meet an enzyme. Almost the same thing happens when you wash clothes. The detergent acts as an emulsifer to dissolve the grease, molecule by molecule, suspending it in water so that it can be rinsed away.

Enzymes break the fat down into fatty acids, which then cross the membrane of the intestine where they are resynthesized back into fats. The newly reformed fats combine with a special type of protein so that they can be picked up by the lymphatic system and carried to the liver (the primary site of metabolism) for further processing. From there, the fat is released into the bloodstream where it can be picked up by fat cells and easily stored as bodyfat.

As you can see, many complex reactions are involved in the digestion and absorption of LCTs. It is a different story with medium chain triglycerides, though. Unlike LCTs, MCTs are more water soluble. With their shorter chain structure, they can be absorbed more easily through the intestinal wall, requiring fewer enzymes or bile salts. An enzyme in the intestinal wall breaks MCTs down into medium chain fatty acids (MCFAs), which then bind with albumin, a water-soluble protein in the blood.

From there, MCTs go right into the bloodstream via the portal vein and are transported to the liver where, inside the cells, they are rapidly oxidized or burned up. In fact, MCT oil is burned so quickly that its calories are turned into body heat – a process known as thermogenesis which boosts the metabolic rate by increasing oxygen consumption. Because very little MCT leaves the liver, MCTs rarely end up being stored as bodyfat.

Researchers at the University of Rochester observed the relationship between MCTs and metabolic rate by comparing the effects of MCT- and LCT-supplemented meals on seven men. In the study, metabolic rate increased 12 percent over six hours after the subjects ate the MCT meals but increased only 4 percent after LCTs were consumed. The results show that MCTs are burned faster than LCTs and boost the metabolism more.[3]

Fats at the Cellular Level

All fats – dietary fats as well as bodyfat – are an energy source for the body. Energy from fats (as well as from carbohydrates and protein) is released from inside cells by the mitochondria, the cell's power plant. But to be released, fats must first enter this power plant. LCTs cannot get in without an escort – a special transport system called the carnitine shuttle.

The shuttle does not run if carbohydrates are being metabolized inside the mitochondria. Consequently, LCTs are barred from entry and cannot be burned for energy – so they may wind up as stored bodyfat.

Unlike LCTs, MCTs do not need an escort to get inside the mitochondria. Instead, they simply diffuse across the mitochondrial membrane. Once inside the mitochondria, MCTs are burned as energy. MCTs can get in even when carbohydrates are there. So, in the presence of carbohydrates, MCTs are burned for energy – another reason why they are not easily stored as bodyfat. Additionally, the burning of MCTs in the mitochondria makes more carbohydrates available for energy, thus increasing endurance and stamina.

MCTs boost energy in another manner. During a series of energy-producing reactions inside the mitochondria, a large portion of MCTs is converted into ketones, which are by-products of fat metabolism. If not excreted, ketones are used by skeletal muscle for fuel – a process that also spares carbohydrates for more sustained energy.

MCTs also spare protein. In a recent study at Calgary University in Alberta, Canada, healthy adults were placed on a low-carbohydrate diet supplemented with MCT oil. The researchers measured the turnover of fat and protein in the subjects' bodies and found that there was an increase in bodyfat burned and a decrease in muscle protein burned for energy. The findings suggest that MCTs help preserve lean mass by inhibiting its breakdown.[4]

Using MCT Oil to Burn Bodyfat

Substituting MCT oil for starchy carbohydrates in the diet can facilitate fat-burning. The reason is that when you reduce your intake of carbohydrates, you suppress the release of insulin. Its antagonist, glucagon, can then go to work. As I explained in Chapter 3, glucagon is the hormone that unlocks bodyfat stores so that they can be used for energy. At the same time, MCT oil keeps your metabolism high, and a high metabolism is conducive to losing bodyfat.

The substitution of MCT oil for carbohydrates should be done only in certain situations, however. In the next chapter, I explain how to properly use MCT oil in your daily food plan to accelerate your bodyfat loss even more – particularly if you have an extremely slow metabolism.

MCT oil should be taken with food and can be poured over vegetables. You can also cook or bake with MCT oil just as you would with any other vegetable oil. Keep the heat at 350 degrees or lower, however, because MCT oil smokes at high temperatures. IMPORTANT: *Do not store MCT oil in anything other than a glass container. It tends to soften containers made of certain types of plastic.*

Gradually introduce MCT oil into your diet at the rate of a few teaspoons a day. This supplement is so rapidly absorbed that it tends to cause stomach cramping if too much is taken at one time or on an empty stomach.

As with any supplement, you should consult your physician before taking MCT oil. This is especially true for diabetics or individuals with a condition called ketosis. **Also, do not use MCT oil or any other supplement on a long-term basis without the guidance of your physician, clinical nutritionist, or registered dietitian.**

❦ *Key Points*

• You need essential fatty acids (EFAs) in your diet to maintain cellular health, to mobilize fat (including cholesterol), and to manufacture prostaglandins, hormone-like substances that are involved in nearly every system in your body.

• Fats are either saturated or unsaturated, and there are two types of unsaturated fats: monounsaturated and polyunsaturated. Unsaturated fats provide EFAs.

• EFA deficiencies typically show up as dry, flaky skin and stiff, painful joints.

• Each day, add one teaspoon of an EFA source to your diet. Good sources include safflower oil, canola oil, flaxseed oil, linseed oil, Evening Primrose oil, and Hain All-Blend.

• On the Lean Bodies program, 10 percent of your total daily food intake comes from fats.

• MCT oil is a remarkable dietary fat that, unlike conventional fats, is rarely stored as bodyfat.

• MCT oil provides a source of energy, helps boost the metabolism, and can be used to help burn bodyfat.

• MCT oil does not provide essential fatty acids and should be used in addition to your EFAs such as safflower or canola oils.

5

❦ *A Leaner Body in Just Seven Weeks*

NOW THAT YOU UNDERSTAND the nutritional aspects of the Lean Bodies program, it is time to put them into action with a seven-week plan designed to shed bodyfat and drop pounds. But first, you need to have your bodyfat measured.

Unlike most "diets," this program does not rely entirely on scales to measure fat loss. Scales take into account too many variables, including water weight gain, and are less accurate than other methods. If you want a true picture of your bodyfat loss, you must have your body composition measured. This measurement gives you the ratio of lean mass (muscle) to bodyfat. I suggest that you have a bodyfat analysis done before you start this program and at the end of your first seven weeks on the program.

There are three accurate methods for determining body composition:

Hydrostatic Underwater Weighing. A sophisticated test for measuring bodyfat, this method uses a large tank of water or swimming pool, a scale with a chair, and a trained technician. Many universities, laboratories, and sports medicine centers offer underwater weighing for a fee.

To obtain your bodyfat measurement, you are first weighed on a scale. Then you are immersed under water while expelling all air from your lungs – since air would make you lighter. Your weight under water is taken, and this measurement is used to calculate your bodyfat using a standard formula.

Ultrasound. Requiring about 10 minutes of time, this method tests three areas on your body. Be sure that the tester uses an FDA-approved analyzer. According to research by Greg Ellis, Ph.D., there is less error when measuring subcutaneous (under the skin) fat with ultrasound than with skinfold calipers, a method explained below. Accuracy for ultrasound is ± 3.2 for men and ± 3.4 for women.

Skinfold Calipers. If you do not have access to ultrasound, another way to determine how much bodyfat you are carrying is to measure skinfold thicknesses using a device called skinfold calipers. With calipers, measurements are taken at specific points on the body. Some systems take three measurements; others, up to nine or more (see Appendix C for the system I recommend). The measurements are then recorded and converted to a bodyfat percentage using a formula. To help ensure accuracy, it is important to use the same technician each time you have this measurement taken.

Food Combining for Constant Energy

As I have explained, you should eat lean proteins, starchy carbohydrates, and lean, fibrous vegetables – with a teaspoon a day of essential fatty acids. Equally important is that these foods be combined properly so that your meals produce a slow release of glucose to keep your energy level high throughout the day.

Each meal should consist of a lean protein, one or two starchy carbohydrates, and one or two lean, fibrous vegetables. By combining complex carbohydrates, high fiber vegetables, and protein at the same meal, you automatically slow-release glucose because the digestive system takes longer to break down this combination of foods. The fiber, in particular, prevents glucose from entering the bloodstream too quickly. This manner of food combining will minimize your hunger and maximize your energy.

During the first two weeks on the program, you should write down all the foods you eat and calculate the nutrient content of your meals, using a guide available in book stores or the *Composition of Foods, Agriculture Handbook No.8*, which is published by the United States Department of Agriculture. Or you can also consult Appendix D, which contains food values for most of the foods you eat on the Lean Bodies program. (The values are taken from *Agriculture Handbook No. 8.*) These guides will help you make sure you are getting enough calories as well as the right balance of nutrients. There is a sample sheet for you to follow on the next page.

The Lean Bodies "Mock Meal"

Spreading your calories throughout the day is an effective way to burn bodyfat and stay energized. As I have mentioned, you eat five meals a day on this program. Two of these meals can be "mini-meals" of protein and starchy carbohydrates or "mock meals," consisting of a carbohydrate/protein drink mixed with water.

To prepare your mock meal, mix two ounces of a carbohydrate supplement with water. We recommend ProCarb™, which is a high quality carbohydrate and protein formulation. This product contains the ingredient "maltodextrin," a starchy carbohydrate manufactured from corn. It has none of the allergy-producing properties found in grains. Like other starchy carbohydrates, maltodextrin is broken down slowly in the body, providing a slow, steady release of energy for about two to three hours after you take it. Appendix C contains a list of other recommended carbohydrate supplements. To make your mock meal taste even better, try flavoring it with Crystal Light drink mix or sugar-free Tang.

For extra protein, you can add an ounce of protein powder to your mock meal. Be sure to keep a good protein powder on hand.

Lean Bodies Program Daily Menu

Date _____

FOOD	QTY.	CALORIES	PROTEIN (Grams)	FAT (Grams)	CARBS (Grams)	SODIUM (Mg)	POTASSIUM (Mg)
Breakfast							
1							
2							
3							
4							
5							
6							
7							
Mock Meal / Mini-Meal							
1							
2							
3							
4							
5							
6							
7							
Lunch							
1							
2							
3							
4							
5							
6							
7							
Mock Meal / Mini-Meal							
1							
2							
3							
4							
5							
6							
7							
Dinner							
1							
2							
3							
4							
5							
6							
7							

When shopping for a protein powder, check the product label to make sure that the supplement contains no added fructose, other sugars, or fillers. The best protein powders are those made from egg or milk protein and fortified with crystalline free form amino acids. A one-ounce scoop of protein powder is used in each mock meal. Refer to Appendix C for a list of recommended protein powders.

People on the program love the simplicity of the mock meals – but there is more to it than that. They come to rely on the sustaining lift it gives them throughout the day. Ken R., for example, had a severe case of low blood sugar (hypoglycemia). "When my blood sugar dropped, I'd become a complete jerk," he says. "And I'd fall asleep after a large meal."

Ken began eating six meals a day, including his mock meals, and upped his calories. Now his hypoglycemia is under control, and he has reduced his bodyfat percentage from 19.8 to 16 percent. "I've become completely 'addicted' to mock meals, and the program itself has totally changed my life."

Nancy M. suffers from chronic fatigue syndrome (CFS), a debilitating disorder that affects as many as 5 million Americans. She says that the multiple meals approach to eating, with the mock meals, is helping to restore her energy levels while she recovers from CFS. "I've made a lifestyle change. I've even started to jog – and that's something I thought I'd never be able to do."

The mock meal is not intended to replace any of your three regular meals – only to supplement them. Mock meals provide extra protein and carbohydrates, help extend energy throughout the day, and represent a source of additional calories so you can gradually up your caloric intake.

Lean Bodies Meal Planning – Program I

The first week, start out by following my basic meal plan. Each week afterwards, add calories to the meal plan. The sample meal plans show you how to do this. As you continue on the program, you will have to make the necessary caloric adjustments according to how active you are. A person who exercises every day or works in a physically demanding profession, for example, will require more calories than will a less active individual.

The basic meal plan, with its subsequent addition of calories, is called Program I. In the next chapter, you learn how to accelerate your bodyfat loss with Programs II and III.

What follows are sample Program I meal plans (one sample meal for each week for seven weeks) for men and for women. These meal plans show you how to gradually increase calories from week to week. Typically, women increase calories by 100; men, by 200. Please note that the men's menus offer examples of how to gradually incorporate MCT oil into your meals. The same gradual increases can be used in the women's menus too.

Additionally, each meal plan provides nutrients in the ratio of: protein, 25 percent; carbohydrates, 65 percent; and fat, 10 percent. Unlike most diets, Lean Bodies daily meal plans provide a potassium/sodium ratio of at least 6-to-1. This helps maintain the body's water balance and is the correct ratio for heart health. If you are concerned about calcium intake, please note that these meal plans provide ample calcium to meet daily requirements. Taking a mineral supplement helps ensure against deficiencies of calcium and other nutrients. Do not forget to take a teaspoon a day of essential fatty acids. Also, be sure to eat every three hours.

PROGRAM I: Women*

Week One Sample Day: 1,500+ Calories

Breakfast

Corn grits (cook 4 tbsp. according to package directions)

3 large scrambled egg whites with ½ tbsp. mild picante sauce

½ tbsp. MCT oil

Mock Meal

2 scoops (2 oz.) carbohydrate supplement mixed with water,
    Crystal Light, or sugar-free Tang

Lunch

3 oz. chicken breast

Brown rice (cook ⅓ cup of rice to yield proper cooked portion)

2 cups broccoli

½ cup peas

Mini-Meal

4 oz. non-fat yogurt

4 rice cakes

Dinner

3 oz. baked cod, 8 oz. potato, 2 cups kale

Salad of 1 cup shredded Romaine lettuce, ½ cup chopped tomato,
    and ½ cup shredded carrots

TOTAL DAILY NUTRIENTS: 1,539 calories; 95.1 g protein; 263.8 g carbohydrate; 9.9 g fat; 722 mg sodium; 3,652 mg potassium; and 752 mg calcium. Note: If you require a specific daily amount of calcium, ask your physician if it may be obtained by increased dairy, deep green leafy vegetables and/or a calcium/magnesium supplement.

The nutrient values of menus are based on use of Pro-Carb™ (protein/carbohydrate supplement) and Hi-Protein Powder™ (protein powder), manufactured by Parrillo Performance. Use of other supplements may yield different nutrient values.

Week Two Sample Day: 1,600+ Calories

Breakfast
3 egg whites
Brown rice (cook ⅓ cup rice to yield proper cooked portion)

Mock Meal
2 scoops (2 oz.) carbohydrate supplement mixed with water,
    Crystal Light, or sugar-free Tang

Lunch
4 oz. baked cod
Brown rice (cook ⅓ cup of rice to yield proper cooked portion)
½ cup black-eyed peas
½ cup squash

Mini-Meal
4 rice cakes
1 scoop (1 oz.) carbohydrate supplement

Dinner
4 oz. baked chicken breast
10 oz. potato
1 cup broccoli
1 cup turnip greens

TOTAL DAILY NUTRIENTS: 1,616 calories; 108.2 g protein; 291.3 g carbohydrate; 8.3 g fat; 543 mg sodium; 3,677 mg potassium; and 555 mg calcium. Note:
If you require a specific daily amount of calcium, ask your physician if it may be
obtained by increased dairy, deep green leafy vegetables and/or a calcium/
magnesium supplement.

Week Three Sample Day: 1,700+ Calories

Breakfast
Oatmeal (cook 8 tbsp. according to package directions)
4 large scrambled egg whites with 2 tbsp. mild picante sauce

Mock Meal
2 scoops (2 oz.) carbohydrate supplement mixed with water,
    Crystal Light, or sugar-free Tang

Lunch
3 oz. baked chicken breast
8 oz. potato
2 cups broccoli
½ cup pinto beans

Mini-Meal
8 oz. non-fat yogurt
4 rice cakes

Dinner
3 oz. baked cod
1 cup cauliflower
Brown rice (cook ⅓ cup to yield proper portion)
1 cup collard greens

TOTAL DAILY NUTRIENTS: 1,739 calories; 110.4 g protein; 292.8 g carbohydrate; 17.7 g fat; 696 mg sodium; 4,309 mg potassium; and 889 mg calcium.
Note: If you require a specific daily amount of calcium, ask your physician if it may
be obtained by increased dairy, deep green leafy vegetables and/or a calcium/
magnesium supplement.

Week Four Sample Day: 1,800+ Calories

Breakfast
Corn grits (cook 8 tbsp. according to package directions)
1 scoop (1 oz.) carbohydrate supplement
1 cup skim milk

Mock Meal
2 scoops (2 oz.) carbohydrate supplement mixed with water,
    Crystal Light, or sugar-free Tang

Lunch
4 oz. chicken
6 oz. potato
2 cups broccoli

Mock Meal
2 scoops (2 oz.) carbohydrate supplement mixed with water,
    Crystal Light, or sugar-free Tang

Dinner
4 oz. turkey breast
2 cups cauliflower
¾ brown rice
2 cups kale

TOTAL DAILY NUTRIENTS: 1,798 calories; 115.4 g protein; 317.7.6 g carbohydrate; 8.4 g fat; 661 mg sodium; 4,058 mg potassium; and 1,038 mg calcium.
Note: If you require a specific daily amount of calcium, ask your physician if it may
be obtained by increased dairy, deep green leafy vegetables and/or a calcium/
magnesium supplement.

Week Five Sample Day: 1,900+ Calories

Breakfast
1 cup oatmeal

Mock Meal
2 scoops (2 oz.) carbohydrate supplement mixed with water,
    Crystal Light, or sugar-free Tang
2 rice cakes

Lunch
3 oz. chicken breast
10 oz. potato
2 cups broccoli
Brown rice (cook ⅓ cup to yield proper portion)

Mock Meal
2 scoops (2 oz.) carbohydrate supplement mixed with water,
    Crystal Light, or sugar-free Tang

Dinner
3 oz. cod
Salad of 1 cup shredded Romaine lettuce, ½ cup chopped tomato,
    and ½ cup shredded carrots
1 cup collard greens

TOTAL DAILY NUTRIENTS: 1,894 calories; 113.4 g protein; 336.6 g carbohydrate; 14.9 g fat; 568 mg sodium; 4,618 mg potassium; and 1,050 mg calcium. Note: If you require a specific daily amount of calcium, ask your physician if it may be obtained by increased dairy, deep green leafy vegetables and/or a calcium/magnesium supplement.

Week Six Sample Day: 2,000+ Calories

Breakfast
1 cup puffed kasha
1 scoop (1 oz.) protein powder mixed in 1 cup skim milk

Mini-Meal
2 corn tortillas
½ cup rice
½ cup pinto beans

Lunch
4 oz. turkey breast
10 oz. potato
2 cups broccoli
1 cup black-eyed peas

Mock Meal
2 scoops (2 oz.) carbohydrate supplement mixed with water,
    Crystal Light, or sugar-free Tang

Dinner
3 large scrambled egg whites
12 oz. potato
10 oz. peas
1 cup turnip greens

TOTAL DAILY NUTRIENTS: 2,015 calories; 124.6 g protein; 369.5 g carbohydrate; 5.7 g fat; 905 mg sodium; 6,046 mg potassium; and 1,320 mg calcium.
Note: If you require a specific daily amount of calcium, ask your physician if it may
be obtained by increased dairy, deep green leafy vegetables and/or a calcium/
magnesium supplement.

Week Seven Sample Day: 2,100+ Calories

Breakfast

1 cup oatmeal

3 large scrambled egg whites

1 cup skim milk

Mock Meal

2 scoops (2 oz.) carbohydrate supplement mixed with water,
    Crystal Light, or sugar-free Tang

Lunch

4 oz. red snapper

12 oz. sweet potato

1 cup lima beans

1½ cups kale

Mock Meal

2 scoops (2 oz.) carbohydrate supplement mixed with water,
    Crystal Light, or sugar-free Tang

Dinner

4 oz. chicken breast

12 oz. potato

2 cups broccoli

2 cups corn

TOTAL DAILY NUTRIENTS: 2,109 calories; 131.3 g protein; 374.2 g carbohydrate; 13.9 g fat; 941 mg sodium; 6,086 mg potassium; and 1,085 mg calcium.
Note: If you require a specific daily amount of calcium, ask your physician if it may
be obtained by increased dairy, deep green leafy vegetables and/or a calcium/
magnesium supplement.

PROGRAM I: Men*

Week One Sample Day: 2,300+ Calories

Breakfast
1 cup oatmeal
6 oz. non-fat yogurt
1 tbsp. MCT oil

Mini-Meal
2 corn tortillas
½ cup rice
½ cup pinto beans

Lunch
6 oz. chicken
Brown rice (cook ⅔ cup to yield proper cooked portion)
1 cup lima beans
1 cup green beans

Mock Meal
2 scoops (2 oz.) carbohydrate supplement and 1 scoop (1 oz.) protein powder
    mixed with water, Crystal Light, or sugar-free Tang

Dinner
4 oz. halibut, 10 oz. potato, 1 cup green beans, 1½ cup kale

TOTAL DAILY NUTRIENTS: 2,308 calories; 134.6 g protein; 373.1 g carbohydrate; 19.0 g fat; 837 mg sodium; 5,424 mg potassium; and 807 mg calcium. Note: If you require a specific daily amount of calcium, ask your physician if it may be obtained by increased dairy, deep green leafy vegetables and/or a calcium/magnesium supplement.

The nutrient values of menus are based on use of Pro-Carb™ (protein/carbohydrate supplement) and Hi-Protein Powder™ (protein powder), manufactured by Parrillo Performance. Use of other supplements may yield different nutrient values.

Week Two Sample Day: 2,500+ Calories

Breakfast
1 cup oatmeal
3 large scrambled egg whites
1 cup skim milk
1 tbsp. MCT oil

Mock Meal
2 scoops (2 oz.) carbohydrate supplement mixed with water,
    Crystal Light, or sugar-free Tang

Lunch
4 oz. tuna
Brown rice (cook ⅔ cup to yield proper cooked portion)
1 cup black-eyed peas
1 cup broccoli

Mini-Meal
2 corn tortillas
½ cup rice (cooked)
½ cup pinto beans

Dinner
5 oz. turkey breast
16 oz. potato
2 cups green beans
2 cups broccoli

TOTAL DAILY NUTRIENTS: 2,533 calories; 159.0 g protein; 413.3 g carbohydrate; 14.7 g fat; 872 mg sodium; 6,190 mg potassium; and 832 mg calcium. Note: If you require a specific daily amount of calcium, ask your physician if it may be obtained by increased dairy, deep green leafy vegetables and/or a calcium/magnesium supplement.

Week Three Sample Day: 2,700+ Calories

Breakfast
4 large scrambled egg whites
14 oz. potato
1 cup skim milk
2 tbsp. MCT oil

Mock Meal
2 scoops (2 oz.) carbohydrate supplement mixed with water,
    Crystal Light, or sugar-free Tang

Lunch
6 oz. turkey breast
12 oz. potato
1 cup green beans
½ cup corn

Mini-Meal
2 corn tortillas
½ cup rice
½ cup pinto beans

Dinner
8 oz. shrimp
Brown rice (cook 1 cup to yield proper cooked portion)
3 cups broccoli
1 cup corn

TOTAL DAILY NUTRIENTS: 2,771 calories; 167.2 g protein; 443.9 g carbohydrate; 11.6 g fat; 1,137 mg sodium; 6,839 mg potassium; and 860 mg calcium. Note: If you require a specific daily amount of calcium, ask your physician if it may be obtained by increased dairy, deep green leafy vegetables and/or a calcium/magnesium supplement.

Week Four Sample Day: 2,900+ Calories

Breakfast
1 cup oatmeal
4 large scrambled egg whites
4 oz. non-fat yogurt
1 tbsp. MCT oil

Mock Meal
2 scoops (2 oz.) carbohydrate supplement mixed with water, Crystal
    Light, or sugar-free Tang

Lunch
6 oz. chicken
8 oz. sweet potato
2 cups corn
1½ cups turnip greens
2 tbsp. MCT oil

Mini Meal
2 corn tortillas
½ cup rice
½ cup pinto beans

Dinner
6 oz. turkey breast
Brown rice (cook ⅔ cup to yield proper cooked portion)
1 cup black-eyed peas
1 cup squash

TOTAL DAILY NUTRIENTS: 2,920 calories; 173.4 g protein; 436.3 g carbohydrate; 21.7 g fat; 814 mg sodium; 4,898 mg potassium; and 851 mg calcium. Note:
If you require a specific daily amount of calcium, ask your physician if it may be
obtained by increased dairy, deep green leafy vegetables and/or a calcium/
magnesium supplement.

Week Five Sample Day: 3,100+ Calories

Breakfast
Barley grits (cook 3 oz. dry grits to yield proper portion)
3 large scrambled egg whites
2 scoops (2 oz.) of carbohydrate supplement
1 tbsp. MCT oil

Mini-Meal
2 oz. tuna
10 oz. potato
4 oz. non-fat yogurt

Lunch
4 oz. chicken
Brown rice (cook ⅔ cup to yield proper portion)
2 cups corn
2 cups broccoli
1 tbsp. MCT oil

Mock Meal
2 scoops (2 oz.) carbohydrate supplement and 1 scoop (1 oz.) protein
powder mixed with water, Crystal Light, or sugar-free Tang

Dinner
2 scoops (2 oz.) of carbohydrate supplement
6 oz. haddock
16 oz. sweet potato
Salad of 1 cup shredded Romaine lettuce, ½ cup chopped tomato,
    ½ cup shredded carrots, and 1 tbsp. MCT oil
1 cup turnip greens

TOTAL DAILY NUTRIENTS: 3,174 calories; 180.4 g protein; 545 g carbohydrate; 12.7 g fat; 974 mg sodium; 5,947 mg potassium; and 1,312 mg calcium. Note:
If you require a specific daily amount of calcium, ask your physician if it may be
obtained by increased dairy, deep green leafy vegetables and/or a calcium/
magnesium supplement.

Week Six Sample Day: 3,300 Calories

Breakfast
Corn grits (cook 4 oz. to yield proper portion)
4 large scrambled egg whites with 2 tbsp. mild picante sauce
2 tbsp. MCT oil

Mock Meal
2 scoops (2 oz.) carbohydrate supplement mixed with water,
    Crystal Light, or sugar-free Tang

Lunch
8 oz. chicken breast
16 oz. potato
2 cups broccoli
1 cup lima beans
2 tbsp. MCT oil

Mini-Meal
2 corn tortillas
½ cup rice
½ cup pinto beans

Dinner
8 oz. cod
2 cups cauliflower
Brown rice (cook 1 cup to yield proper cooked portion)
1½ cups kale
1 tbsp. MCT oil

TOTAL DAILY NUTRIENTS: 3,299 calories; 176.2 g protein; 500.3 g carbohydrate; 11.9 g fat; 1,192 mg sodium; 6,739 mg potassium; and 929 mg calcium. Note: If you require a specific daily amount of calcium, ask your physician if it may be obtained by increased dairy, deep green leafy vegetables and/or a calcium/magnesium supplement.

Week Seven Sample Day: 3,500 Calories

Breakfast
1 cup oatmeal
3 large scrambled egg whites
1 cup skim milk
1 tbsp. MCT oil

Mock Meal
2 scoops (2 oz.) carbohydrate supplement mixed with water,
    Crystal Light, or sugar-free Tang

Lunch
6 oz. chicken breast
16 oz. sweet potato
1 cup black-eyed peas
1 cup squash
1 tbsp. MCT oil

Mock Meal
2 scoops (2 oz.) carbohydrate supplement and 1 scoop (1 oz.) protein
powder mixed with water, Crystal Light, or sugar-free Tang

Dinner
2 scoops (2 oz.) carbohydrate supplement
4 oz. turkey
Brown rice (cook ⅔ cup to yield proper cooked portion)
2 cups corn
2 cups green beans
2 tbsp. MCT oil

TOTAL DAILY NUTRIENTS: 3,497 calories; 186.3 g protein; 536.3 g carbohydrate; 16.8 g fat; 1,014 mg sodium; 6,210 mg potassium; and 1,221 mg calcium.
Note: If you require a specific daily amount of calcium, ask your physician if it may
be obtained by increased dairy, deep green leafy vegetables and/or a calcium/
magnesium supplement.

Your Lean Bodies Shopping List

To help get you started, here is a sample shopping list that covers one week of the program for one person. For convenience and variety, I have included both frozen and fresh foods.

Lean Proteins

2 dozen eggs (Buy eggs that are on sale because the yolks are smaller and the whites are larger.)

2 lbs. sliced turkey breast or whole turkey breast

8 whole chicken breasts, skinless

½ lb. cod

½ lb. halibut

2 6-oz. cans water-packed tuna and/or 4 3 ½-oz. cans water-packed tuna (These make convenient mini-meals.)

Starchy Carbohydrates

18-oz. box old-fashioned oatmeal (not instant or quick cooking) or other whole grain cereal

14-oz. package brown rice

16-oz. package frozen green peas

16-oz. package frozen corn

16-oz. package frozen lima beans

2-4 potatoes or sweet potatoes

Lean, Fibrous Vegetables

16-oz. package frozen green beans

16-oz. package carrots

2 bags fresh kale

2 heads fresh broccoli

2 heads fresh cauliflower

16-oz. package frozen zucchini

1 head Romaine or red-leafed lettuce

An ample supply of fresh salad vegetables such as onions,
tomatoes, green peppers, cucumbers, radishes, and so forth

Fats

1 32-oz. bottle of oil (safflower oil, canola oil, flaxseed oil,
linseed oil, or Hain All-Blend)

MCT oil

1 can of non-stick spray

Spices and condiments

No-salt seasoning mix

Cider vinegar

Paprika

Garlic powder

Onion powder

Italian seasoning

Molly McButter in various flavors (This seasoning tastes
just like butter and is great on vegetables.)

Dairy

1 quart skim milk

Non-fat yogurt

Lean Cooking in Bulk

Once you understand how to plan your meals, the next important lesson on the Lean Bodies program is learning how to cook in bulk – preparing large quantities of food for the week ahead. This further simplifies the program, saves time, and makes meal preparation a breeze. Many people do their bulk cooking on Sunday night for convenience. Here are several tips to help you:

1. Cook large quantities of lean proteins and refrigerate or freeze some for future use.

2. Chop up large quantities of salad vegetables and place them in a crisper. When you are ready for your next salad, it is right there in your refrigerator.

3. Cook a large pot of brown rice and then refrigerate it for the week ahead. When you are ready to eat it, simply pop it in the microwave.

4. Hard boil eggs ahead of time and refrigerate them. When you are ready to eat them, discard the yolks.

5. When making one of our Lean Bodies recipes (see Appendix B), such as a soup, casserole, or chili, increase the recipe, making enough for two, four, or six meals. Soups and chilies freeze wonderfully. Extra casseroles may be frozen unbaked for future baking or baked ahead for future defrosting and heating.

6. For extra convenience, package soups and chilies in single-serving portions. Freeze these foods in small, round, thin containers rather than in large, tall, rectangular containers. Food frozen in this manner defrosts much more efficiently.

Food Preparation

Your freezer is your best friend in meal preparation for convenience, nutritional value, time savings, money savings, and great tasting meals.

Here are 10 tips for freezing food:

1. Select only the best quality – and freshest – foods for freezing.

2. Prepare fresh food for freezing as soon as possible after gathering or purchasing.

3. Cooked foods should be cooled to room temperature or refrigerated before freezing.

4. Use airtight wrapping bags and containers designed for freezing. Double bagging prolongs the freezer life of delicate foods such as asparagus, tomatoes, herbs, and spices.

5. Label and date each frozen item.

6. Using a freezer thermometer, periodically check your freezer temperature to make sure it maintains the proper storage temperature of zero degrees.

7. Foods that have been frozen too long will fade or change colors. Vegetables will become limp when cooked. Gray and white spots on food or dried edges on food are signs of freezer burn – a result of poor wrapping or storage in non-airtight containers.

8. To avoid spoilage, thaw food in the refrigerator or defrost in your microwave oven prior to cooking or serving. Discard any defrosted food that appears spoiled or has an off-color.

9. Never refreeze food that has been completely thawed. Make sure that fish and poultry you plan to freeze is fresh. If food has been previously frozen (like many fish items), be sure to cook it before you refreeze it.

10. Undercook foods slightly if you are planning to freeze them. If you do not, overcooking can occur during reheating.

Do not forget to try the Lean Bodies recipes in Appendix B. This special section includes many delicious dishes, from oven fried potatoes to spaghetti. *Bon appetit!*

Eating Out – the Lean Way

Ron S., age 36, had been a dieter ever since he was a teenager. But no matter what diet he went on, he always gained the weight back. Ron heard about Lean Bodies on the radio and decided to give it a try.

One of the first things that struck him about the program was that he could easily eat in restaurants – something he enjoys. Today, 11 pounds lighter, Ron says, "Before now, I had always been eating with guilt. With this program, I have permission to eat – even in restaurants."

In today's on-the-move society, many of us dine out – more so for convenience than for luxury. On the Lean Bodies program, you can eat in most restaurants. (See Appendix E for a list of restaurants that serve meals you can eat on the Lean Bodies program.) The first rule of thumb is to identify restaurants that offer fish and chicken entrees, salad bars, vegetables, baked potatoes, rice, and other foods on the program. Calling ahead is a good way to find out what meals are available and how they are prepared.

People on the Lean Bodies program become masters at another important rule of dining out: learning how to "special order." For example:

• If fish and chicken entrees come fried, ask that they be baked or broiled instead – without oil.

• Request that vegetables be steamed or microwaved.

• In Oriental restaurants, order chicken and fish dishes without sauces.

• Order oil and vinegar salad dressings or order salad dressing on the side.

• Request that no fats be added to the food.

Actually, you will be able to eat out at restaurants quite easily on the Lean Bodies program. That's one of the beauties of this system – it lets you lead a normal social life. No watching others eat real food while you have only a liquid shake. No bringing along your own salad dressing or other inconvenient items, as you have to with many diet programs. Just order carefully, and you should have no trouble staying on the Lean Bodies program in restaurants.

But, to make it even easier, some restaurants now offer Lean Bodies meals right on their menus. The quiet revolution began with Tong's, a Chinese restaurant located in North Dallas, who asked me to help them develop a "lean" section in their menu. Next, Cheddar's, a local chain, wished to offer a Lean Bodies Plate to their customers. From there everything snowballed: an executive from a national chain, The Black-Eyed Pea restaurants, attended one of my weight-loss clinics here in Dallas. He was so impressed with this radical new approach to eating to *lose* weight that he worked to interest the company's president in featuring Lean Bodies meals on The Black-Eyed Pea menu. I worked closely with the restaurant chain's Research and Development department to ensure that these new Lean Bodies entrees match the protein/carbohydrate/fat ratios you should have on the program. These menu items are now available in all The Black-Eyed Pea restaurants. There are currently over a hundred The Black-Eyed Pea restaurants, both company and franchise, located throughout the country and that number is predicted to double by the year 1996.

Other restaurants soon expressed interest, and we were able to develop Lean Bodies meals to be offered on the menus of participating Bonanza* restaurants, Cheddars, Pulido's and Two Pesos. Following are some examples of the types of Lean Bodies meals you can order at these restaurants**:

---

*Not all Bonanza restaurants participate in the Lean Bodies program. Please check with your local restaurant before planning your outing.

**Cliff Sheats' Lean Bodies meals are a part of a Cliff Sheats' Lean Bodies promotion, and are subject to change or expiration. Always check with your local Lean Bodies restaurant for participation and updates.

Bonanza

Grilled Chicken Dinner

    6 oz. boneless, skinless chicken breast

    Baked potato (plain)

    Freshtastiks Foodbar (salad, vegetables, low calorie dressing)

Cheddars

Lemon Pepper Chicken

    Grilled chicken breast

    Salad

    Vegetable

Grilled Chicken Salad

    A seasoned boneless, skinless chicken breast, charbroiled and sliced on a bed of fresh salad greens

Salad and Baked Potato

    Dinner salad served with baked potato (plain)

The Black-Eyed Pea

    Charbroiled chicken breast

    Black-eyed peas

    Baked potato (plain)

    Salad

Pulidos

Pollo Prieto

    Mexican-style blackened chicken served with charrabeans and grilled vegetables

Chicken California

   Chicken breast seasoned with garlic sauce, grilled and served
   with steamed squash and salad

Two Pesos

Grilled Chicken Fajita Plate

   1 3½ oz. boneless skinless grilled chicken breast
   3½ oz. rice
   Side salad (lettuce, tomatoes, low calorie dressing)
   2 corn tortillas

Chicken Fajita

   ½ oz. lettuce, ¼ oz. tomatoes and 1¾ oz. grilled chicken
   served in a corn tortilla

Chicken Fajita Salad

   6 oz. lettuce, ½ oz. tomatoes, 3½ oz. grilled chicken served
   with low calorie dressing
   (Shell is whole wheat tortilla, fried – do not eat)

As you can see, the above menu selections are high in nutrition
and taste – and thus perfect for the Lean Bodies program. In addition,
if you dine out with friends and family who want to "indulge" in other
foods, these restaurants have an extensive array of other foods on the
menu. In other words, there is something for everyone.

   In Appendix E, you will find a list of restaurants offering Lean
Bodies meals by area. As the Lean Bodies approach to nutrition
becomes more popular, I expect to see other restaurants offering
similar meals. Keep in mind, too, that some of the restaurants now
listed as participants may not do so permanently, while new restaurants may come on board. So that you can dine out and stay lean, I

want to keep you informed on the restaurants around the country that serve Lean Bodies meals. To get updates on participating restaurants in your area, simply call 1-817-921-3346.

There is no need to worry about your food selections while traveling either. All you have to do is pack your Lean Bodies book. That way, you can easily check the city you are visiting for restaurants serving Lean Bodies meals.

Support

As with most group activities, Lean Bodies classes provide a level of support for those on the program – a decided advantage when you are embarking on a lifestyle change. Most of the case histories I document come from the participants in my Lean Bodies classes. But recently, I heard about Boyce W., 44, who had been overweight most of his life. Like so many others, he had been on and off diets, including a medically supervised fast – all to no avail.

Boyce is a regular listener of "The Weekend Workout," a show hosted by Larry North on KLIF, a popular talk radio station in Dallas. Larry mentions the Lean Bodies program often and is one of our strongest advocates. In addition, I am a regular guest on the radio. Boyce learned about the program by listening to Larry and me on the show, and he decided to try it on his own. In one year, he lost 60 pounds and boosted his energy level, which had fallen considerably as a result of repetitive dieting. "Lean Bodies is now my lifestyle," he says.

For most people, making a lifestyle change is easier if a spouse, family member, or loved one makes the commitment too. Typically, when one family member is successful on the program, others follow. That was the case with Donna and Danny M. As Donna explains, "One day, I looked in the mirror, and said 'No more.' I looked so bad that I didn't want to go anywhere or be with anyone. And I was tired of shopping at fat ladies' stores. Finally, I started Cliff's program, and it was like seeing the light at the end of the tunnel."

Donna reduced her bodyfat considerably on the program – from 27.4 percent to a much leaner percentage – and developed the healthy look of a fitness model. Meanwhile, her husband Danny had been steadily putting on bodyfat, year after year. "After trying every diet, I had reached a point where I didn't know what would work. Donna had gotten great results on Lean Bodies, so I decided to try it."

Danny gradually built his caloric intake up to 3,200 calories a day, while losing between one-and-a-half and three pounds a week. "Before, I had always thought that to lose bodyfat you had to stop eating. No one had ever told me that to lose, you have to eat more."

His decrease in bodyfat pleased him as much as his increases in strength and lean mass. Danny, a businessman, looks so fit that people in the gym where he works out have asked him to be their personal trainer.

"I don't think I could have accomplished this level of fitness without nutrition," he says. "We will absolutely be on this program the rest of our lives."

Fortunately, the Lean Bodies program is one the entire family can live on. Another case in point: Susan B.'s family is excited about foods she now prepares. For nearly 10 years, Susan had followed a macrobiotic diet, which is restricted to vegetables and grains. "My kids hated the food," she told me.

Not only has the Lean Bodies way of eating met with her family's approval, it has also rescued Susan from constant fatigue. "Until now, I could never get through the day without a nap, and I had throat infections constantly. Now my energy has spiralled upward. Also, I reduced my bodyfat from about 22 percent to 18 percent."

❦ *Key Points*

- As you start the Lean Bodies program, have your body composition tested by one of three methods: underwater weighing, ultrasound, or skinfold calipers. Have it tested periodically, and keep track of your scale weight too.

- On the Lean Bodies program, each meal should include a lean protein, one or two starchy carbohydrates, and one or two lean, fibrous vegetables. This method of food combining slow-releases glucose to keep energy levels high throughout the day. And, protein at each meal helps raise your metabolic rate.

- Eat five times a day, including three full meals and two mini-meals of protein and a starchy carbohydrate or two "mock meals" made from a carbohydrate supplement and a protein powder. Be sure to eat every three hours.

- Start with Program I. Gradually increase your calories from week to week. Typically, women increase their calories by 100 each week; men, by 200 calories each week. This varies according to your activity level and metabolic status.

- For convenience, cook your foods in bulk. That way, they will be ready to heat up or microwave during the week.

- While following the Lean Bodies program, you can eat out in most restaurants, once you learn how to order with a little care.

6

CHAPTER SIX ¶ *Accelerating Bodyfat Loss*

EVERYONE BURNS FAT at a different rate, depending on individual characteristics such as sex, age, activity level, and overall metabolic condition. In some cases, the Lean Bodies program should be modified for individuals with slow, fragile metabolisms to "jump start" the fat-burning process or to break plateaus. The modifications include three programs, each designed to maximize your fat-burning potential. The programs are as follows:

Program I

Everyone who begins the Lean Bodies program starts on Program I. Described in the previous chapter, this is the basic food plan that includes lean proteins, starchy carbohydrates, and lean, fibrous vegetables eaten in combination at all meals. You should start with the basic food plan, adding calories each week. Stay on Program I as long as you are losing bodyfat at a steady rate. Unless you hit a plateau, there is no need to make any changes in the way you are eating. Refer to the Program I food plans in Chapter Five to help you with your menu planning.

Program II

If you begin the program with a high percentage of bodyfat, say 30 percent or more, you should move to Program II after two weeks on Program I.

Program II modifies the basic food plan in Program I by excluding starchy carbohydrates from the evening meal. There are good reasons for this. First, by reducing your carbohydrate consumption, you inhibit the release of insulin. This in turn stimulates glucagon, the hormone that helps unlock fat stores.

Second, when starchy carbohydrates are dropped at night, fewer stored carbohydrates (glycogen) are available for energy the next morning. In the absence of glycogen, your body starts burning fatty acids (stored bodyfat) for energy – particularly if you exercise aerobically before breakfast. Fat loss is accelerated as a result. Pre-breakfast aerobics are a great fat loss tool, as Faith Y. found out. By following the Lean Bodies program and exercising on a stationary bike at 5:30 every morning, she reduced her bodyfat content from 40 percent to 28 percent. (She originally started the program to reduce her cholesterol, which at the time was 280. In addition to losing substantial bodyfat, Faith lowered her cholesterol to 201 in six weeks.)

Third, when you eat starchy carbohydrates at breakfast and lunch, they are efficiently synthesized into glycogen for storage in the muscles – and are less likely to be converted to fat.

On Program II, do not eat after 7:00 p.m. If you do feel hungry after that time, eat a lean protein. Use MCT oil to help you burn fat and boost your metabolism.

Stay on Program II for no longer than two or three weeks. When adding starchy carbohydrates back in your evening meal, choose corn, beans, and legumes. These are higher in protein than other starchy carbohydrates and therefore have a higher metabolic effect. Do not forget to take a teaspoon a day of your essential fatty acids.

Here is a sample food plan for Program II, with carbohydrates excluded from the evening meal:

Program II Sample Meal Plan*

Breakfast
3 large scrambled egg whites
10 oz. potato
4 oz. tomato sauce
1 tbsp. MCT oil

Mock Meal
2 scoops (2 oz.) carbohydrate supplement mixed with water,
    Crystal Light, or sugar-free Tang

Lunch
4 oz. tuna
10 oz. sweet potato
1 cup broccoli
1 cup corn

Mini-Meal
8 oz. of non-fat yogurt
4 rice cakes

Dinner
4 oz. chicken breast
Salad of 1 cup shredded Romaine lettuce, ½ cup chopped
    tomatoes, ½ cup shredded carrots, and 2 tbsp. MCT oil
2 cups kale

TOTAL DAILY NUTRIENTS: 1,998 calories; 115.7 g protein; 284.5 g carbohydrate; 12.9 g fat; 652 mg sodium; 4,320 mg potassium; and 889 mg calcium. Note: If you require a specific daily amount of calcium, ask your physician if it may be obtained by increased dairy, deep green leafy vegetables and/or a calcium/magnesium supplement.

The nutrient values of menus are based on use of Pro-Carb™ (protein/carbohydrate supplement) and Hi-Protein Powder™ (protein powder), manufactured by Parrillo Performance. Use of other supplements may yield different nutrient values.

Program III

This program is designed for "chronic dieters" – people who have dieted so long, either on shake fasts or other calorically restricted diets, that their metabolisms are extremely sluggish. You fit this category if you have a history of dieting and are not losing an appreciable amount of bodyfat after three weeks on Program II.

At this level, exclude starchy carbohydrates after 3:00 p.m. to speed up fat loss. Include a daily aerobic workout in your schedule, either in the morning, the evening, or both. Again, your body will be forced to draw on its own stored fat for energy in the absence of enough glycogen. As the food plans below show, calories from lean proteins and lean, fibrous vegetables are still high.

Some people on Program III experience a loss of energy from the exclusion of starchy carbohydrates. If this happens to you, compensate by using MCT oil, taken with food in the afternoon, with mock meals, and in the evening – about one or two tablespoons each time. Used this way, MCT oil acts as a pure energy source because it is absorbed like a carbohydrate; it spares carbohydrate (glycogen); it helps your body enter a fat-burning mode; and it helps speed up your metabolism.

Program III should be followed for no longer than two or three days during any given week and not longer than two or three weeks. When you add starchy carbohydrates back in, stick to those with a higher protein content (corn, beans, and legumes). Do not forget to supplement your meals with a teaspoon a day of your essential fatty acids. And if you feel hungry, eat a lean protein. Remember too that it is always better to increase your activity level through exercise than to decrease calories.

Here is a sample meal plan for Program III:

Program III Sample Meal Plan*

Breakfast
1 cup oatmeal
3 large scrambled egg whites
1 cup skim milk
1 tbsp. MCT oil

Mock Meal
2 scoops (2 oz.) carbohydrate supplement mixed with water,
   Crystal Light, or sugar-free Tang

Lunch
6 oz. turkey breast
16 oz. sweet potato
2 cups green beans
1 tbsp. MCT oil

Mini-Meal
1 scoop (1 oz.) of protein powder mixed with water

Dinner
6 oz. red snapper
2 cups squash
2 cups broccoli
1 tbsp. MCT oil

TOTAL DAILY NUTRIENTS: 2,268 calories; 174.4 g protein; 282.9 g carbohydrate; 13.1 g fat; 785 mg sodium; 4,942 mg potassium; and 1,314 mg calcium. Note: If you require a specific daily amount of calcium, ask your physician if it may be obtained by increased dairy, deep green leafy vegetables and/or a calcium/magnesium supplement.

*The nutrient values of menus are based on use of Pro-Carb™ (protein/carbohydrate supplement) and Hi-Protein Powder™ (protein powder), manufactured by Parrillo Performance. Use of other supplements may yield different nutrient values.

¶ *Key Points*

• In some cases, the Lean Bodies program should be modified to accelerate fat-burning.

• If you hit a plateau, move to Program II of the Lean Bodies program, which excludes starchy carbohydrates from the evening meal. This inhibits the release of insulin and stimulates glucagon, the hormone that helps unlock fat stores. Also, when starchy carbohydrates are excluded in the evening, your body starts drawing on fatty acids (stored bodyfat) for energy in the absence of glycogen from carbohydrates.

• Program III speeds fat loss even more. At this level, you exclude starchy carbohydrates after 3 p.m.

• Use MCT oil on Program Levels II and III to provide extra energy and help your body burn fat.

7

❦ *Vitamins: Metabolic Catalysts*

ALL THE BIOCHEMICAL REACTIONS that go on inside our bodies at the cellular level, from metabolism to growth, depend on vitamins and minerals. Each has its own specific role in the body, yet no vitamin or mineral acts alone. They must all be present in certain amounts to maintain good health. Too much or too little of one or more can create an imbalance, and this can be damaging to your body.

Much is being said today about vitamins and minerals — specifically, whether or not to supplement our diets with them. Increasingly however, more physicians are recommending supplementation. In fact, a very strong case for supplements can be built, if you consider the following:

Dietary deficiencies. Most of our population simply does not eat nutritiously enough to even meet the Recommended Dietary Allowances (RDA)* for vitamins and minerals, according to the Anarem report, a detailed study of three-day dietary records of 21,500 people surveyed in a recent USDA National Food Consumption Survey. The Anarem report revealed the following:[1]

• Only 3 percent of the population ate the recommended number of servings from the four food groups over a three-day period.

• Only 12 percent of the population ate 100 percent of the RDA for protein, calcium, iron, vitamin A, thiamin, riboflavin, and vitamin C.

---

*The RDA are the most commonly accepted guidelines for levels of nutrient intake, although they do not reflect optimal levels of nutrition for the individual. Furthermore, nutrient levels that do not meet the RDA do not necessarily put you at risk of clinical deficiency.

• No one consumed 100 percent of theRDA for vitamin B-6, vitamin B-12, magnesium, protein, calcium, iron, vitamin A, thiamin, riboflavin, and vitamin C.

Low-calorie dieting leads to vitamin and mineral deficiencies as well. One study analyzed 11 popular weight-loss regimens and discovered that every one was low in vital nutrients. The nutrients most often found to be deficient were thiamine, vitamin B-6, calcium, iron, magnesium, and zinc.[2]

According to the Council for Responsible Nutrition, the National Cancer Institute is supporting more than 20 research studies on diet and cancer — at a cost of $27 million. Most of these studies are investigating the potential use of nutritional supplements in the fight against cancer.[3] Citing this and other research supporting the benefit of supplementation, the Council concluded that: "Evidence from several lines of research indicates that, for most people, it makes more sense to follow a healthy lifestyle, eat a healthful diet, and use nutritional supplements regularly than fail to avail themselves of the potential benefits of supplemental use."[4]

Soil depletion. You cannot always rely on the nutrient content in your foods. Modern farming methods, for example, have depleted the soil in many areas of the country, ultimately reducing the nutrients in food. Between 1950 and 1975, according to *Composition of Foods, Agriculture Handbook No. 8* from the U.S. Department of Agriculture, the protein content in a cup of rice dropped nearly 11 percent; calcium, 21 percent; and iron 28.6 percent. Cabbage has always been traditionally high in vitamin C. Now it has zero vitamin C. In 1945, the protein content of wheat was 17 percent; by 1985, it had dropped to 9 percent.[5] Clearly, our foods may not supply all the nutrients we need — so supplementing the diet helps compensate for what is missing.

Absorption and bioavailability. Some nutrients interact in such a way that they block absorption of certain vitamins and minerals. For example, dietary fiber may curb the absorption of iron. A related issue is that of "bioavailability" — how well vitamins and minerals are absorbed from the foods we eat. And many are not well absorbed, including calcium, iron, and chromium.

Loss of nutrients. Exercise causes the body to demand nutrients. B-complex vitamins, calcium, potassium, magnesium, iron — these are a few of the nutrients that can be depleted with vigorous exercise. Nutrients are also lost through perspiration or urine.

Cooking can destroy certain vitamins, particularly vitamins C, A, and pantothenic acid.

Stress is another factor that depletes the nutrients in your body. Suppose you are stuck in traffic, it is 2:30 p.m., and you are late for an important meeting. The entire time, your body is rapidly using up vitamin C and vitamin B-complex. That single stressful situation has just predisposed you to a nutrient-deficient state.

Biochemical individuality. Each of us is quite different, not only in the way we look and act but also in how our bodies require different nutrients. This difference is referred to as "biochemical individuality," a term coined by the late Dr. Roger J. Williams of the University of Texas at Austin, who discovered the B-complex vitamin pantothenic acid and named folic acid. Our own personal nutrient requirements may vary, depending on our level of activity, age, condition, sex, and other factors. Women, for example, may need more calcium and trace minerals than men to help prevent osteoporosis. And athletes may need more protein than non-athletes. No two people are alike in their need for various nutrients.

The point is, nutritional supplementation provides extra insurance that you are giving your body all the resources it needs for optimum health. But as I tell my classes: Do not even think about taking supplements until you are eating the right foods in the right combinations and caloric amounts. Equally important: You do not have to take supplements to be successful on this program.

Before you decide whether or not to take supplements, I think it is important for you to understand the function of certain nutrients in your body, starting with vitamins.

Vitamins

Vitamins assist in the growth of all body tissues and are essential for the release of energy in the body. There are two classifications: water-soluble and fat-soluble. Water-soluble vitamins such as the B-complex vitamins and vitamin C cannot be stored by the body. This is because they do not easily penetrate the lipid-based membranes of cells and therefore must constantly be replenished by the diet. These vitamins are involved primarily in metabolism.

Fat-soluble vitamins such as vitamins A, D, and E act like hormones in the body. Unlike water-soluble vitamins, they can enter cell membranes and are thus easily stored in body tissues.

If you decide to supplement your diet with vitamins, select a brand that contains a wide variety of vitamins and is manufactured by a reputable company. (See Appendix C for a recommended list of products.) Vitamins are food, so take them during or directly after meals because their absorption is improved with food. Always consult your physician before taking any supplement.

Here is a closer look at how the water-soluble and fat-soluble vitamins function in the body.

Vitamin A and Beta Carotene

Vitamin A is a versatile nutrient because it regulates so many essential functions in the body, including immune function. Vitamin A helps fight viral and bacterial infections, possibly by stimulating the activity of white blood cells. Vitamin A also helps tissues heal faster, aids in vision, and keeps the skin healthy. This nutrient has also been shown to have a protective effect against cancer, particularly skin and lung cancer. In large doses, vitamin A is toxic because it accumulates in the liver and other organs. Food sources of vitamin A include eggs and milk.

A nutrient called beta carotene (pro-vitamin A) has received a great deal of attention in scientific circles. It appears to have many therapeutic benefits, including the prevention and treatment of cancer. Studies of large populations have found that the more beta carotene consumed in the diet, the lower the risk of developing certain cancers, including those of the breast, lung, stomach, and mouth. Other studies have shown that high concentrations of beta carotene in the blood are associated with reduced risk of cancer.[6]

Beta carotene's anti-cancer effects may be related to its role in immune function. This nutrient boosts the activity of lymphocytes (white blood cells in the lymphatic system) and increases the number of T-cells (lymphocytes that help other cells destroy invading agents).

Unlike vitamin A, beta carotene does not cause toxicity, even when taken in high doses. This is because beta carotene is converted into vitamin A only as the body needs it. In the diet, beta carotene can be obtained from such foods as carrots; all yellow and orange vegetables; green, leafy vegetables; and broccoli.

B-Complex Vitamins

Vital for energy, B-complex vitamins are involved in nearly every reaction in the body, from the manufacture of new red blood cells to the metabolism of carbohydrates, fat, and protein. Unfortunately, though, cooking and food processing destroy these nutrients, and stress causes deficiencies.

Thiamine or vitamin B₁ was the first member of the B-complex family to be identified and therefore is a well-known nutrient. It plays a key role in the production of energy. In addition, thiamine is essential for the maintenance of a good appetite, normal digestion, and the health of the gastrointestinal tract. It has also been shown to enhance muscular endurance. Yet many people are deficient in this vitamin. Eating foods low in thiamine, cutting calories to lose weight, overcooking foods – these are a few of the practices that cause deficiencies or destroy thiamine in the body.

The best food sources of thiamine are legumes and whole grains. Your requirement for thiamine increases as you get older. It is often difficult to meet requirements for this B vitamin because thiamine is found in a fairly limited range of foods – so taking supplemental thiamine is good insurance. All members of the B-complex family, including thiamine, should be taken together to ensure balance.

Riboflavin (vitamin B₂) is involved in the breakdown and utilization of carbohydrates, fats, and proteins. It plays a role in cellular respiration by working with enzymes in the utilization of cell oxygen. Additionally, riboflavin helps the body absorb iron and maintains the health of mucous membranes.

Riboflavin is found primarily in brewer's yeast and organ meats. Even so, the amount of riboflavin in these foods is quite small; therefore, it is difficult to get all you need without supplementation. Additionally, the more active you are, the more riboflavin you need. Deficiencies typically show up in the skin, usually as cracks at the corner of the mouth. Sensitivity to light is another symptom of a riboflavin deficiency.

Niacin (vitamin B₃) has received a lot of press because of its cholesterol-lowering effect. A certain type of supplemental niacin does lower cholesterol when taken in extremely high doses. In cases like this, niacin is considered to be a drug to be used only under a physician's supervision. Megadoses of niacin can poison the liver.[7]

Niacin is involved in the metabolism of carbohydrate, fat, and protein and is essential for the health of the nervous system, skin, and digestive system. Lean proteins such as chicken, turkey, and fish are excellent sources of niacin. Deficiency symptoms include skin eruptions, fatigue, muscular weakness, and indigestion.

Pantothenic acid is a nutrient you do not hear much about, but this B-complex vitamin has many roles to play in the body. It stimulates the adrenal glands and boosts production of hormones responsible for healthy skin and nerves. Like other B-complex vitamins, it helps release energy from foods. The health of the digestive tract depends on pantothenic acid. It also enhances the body's ability to withstand stress and aids in the prevention of premature aging.

Pantothenic acid is found in all plants and animals. In addition, it can be synthesized in the body by intestinal bacteria – so deficiencies are virtually unknown. Refined and processed foods are devoid of this nutrient, and about a third of the pantothenic acid in meat is destroyed by cooking.

Vitamin B₆ (pyroxidine) is rather amazing because it influences nearly every system in the body. For example, it assists in creating amino acids (the building blocks of protein), turning carbohydrates into glucose, metabolizing fats, producing neurotransmitters (chemicals that relay nerve impulses), and manufacturing antibodies to ward off infection.

Also, vitamin B₆ is needed to prevent the build-up of homocysteine in the blood, a toxic by-product of the amino acid methionine.

Homocysteine causes the cells lining arterial walls to deteriorate. In response, the arteries start rebuilding by creating new cells and new connective tissue that then attract cholesterol and triglycerides. This reconstructive process can eventually lead to atherosclerosis (hardening of the arteries).

Supplemental vitamin B_6 has been used in the treatment of many disorders, including premenstrual tension, carpal tunnel syndrome, and kidney stones. Deficiencies are not common, although certain prescription drugs such as hydralazine (for high blood pressure), penicillin, and theophylline (for asthma) can deplete vitamin B_6 by blocking its action.

If you are active, you may be interested in knowing that extra vitamin B_6 can help boost endurance. Research has demonstrated that supplemental B_6 may improve Vo2 max, a measurement of the body's ability to burn oxygen.[8]

The best food sources of vitamin B_6 include salmon, Atlantic mackerel, white meat chicken, halibut, tuna, broccoli, lentils, and brown rice.

B_{12} (Cobalamin) regulates many functions in the body, as do the other members of the B-complex family. Among the most vital is the production of red blood cells. Vitamin B_{12} is the director in this process, making sure that enough cells are manufactured. Without Vitamin B_{12}, red blood cell production falls off, and the result is misshapen cells and anemia.

Vitamin B_{12} has a partner in the production of red blood cells: folic acid, another B-complex vitamin that regulates a host of functions in the body, including the synthesis of RNA and DNA – the genetic material responsible for cell division. Deficiencies of either vitamin can lead to a condition called megoblastic anemia, in which red blood cells are enlarged, carry less hemoglobin, and have a short life span.

Many diets tend to supply marginal amounts of folic acid, which is abundantly found in dark green, leafy vegetables, cauliflower, meats, and eggs. One reason may be that storage and cooking can destroy as much as 80 percent of the vitamin.

For most people, deficiencies of vitamin B_{12} are rare, as long as a protein-rich diet is followed. Vitamin B_{12} can be obtained only from animal foods, including poultry, fish, eggs, and milk. Strict vegans (people who eat no food of animal origin), however, are candidates for a vitamin B_{12} deficiency. This is also true of people on cholesterol-lowering medication, potassium-replacement agents, anti-ulcer drugs, and anti-convulsants. These can upset the balance of vitamin B_{12} in the body.

Others at risk include people with an inherited inability to absorb the vitamin (a potentially fatal condition called pernicious anemia). Some individuals have trouble absorbing vitamin B_{12} because they lack something called an "intrinsic factor," a molecule produced in the stomach. This molecule binds to vitamin B_{12} and transports it to the intestinal wall to be absorbed.

A serious consequence of vitamin B_{12} deficiency can be irreversible damage to the nervous system. This is because vitamin B_{12} helps build myelin, a protein sheath that envelops your nerves. Nerve tissue degenerates without myelin, causing a host of problems that include numbness, prickly sensations, depression, and memory loss.

Vitamin C

Vitamin C maintains collagen, helps create red blood cells, promotes wound healing, fights bacterial infection, and protects eyes against the oxidative damage that leads to cataracts. And lately, there is mounting interest in vitamin C as a cholesterol fighter. Researchers at the University of Texas Southwestern Medical Center discovered that vitamin C (and vitamin E to a lesser extent) prevented the oxidation of LDL cholesterol – a process caused by free radicals. These are a group of unstable molecules that destroy otherwise healthy cells by robbing them of oxygen. This robbery weakens the immune system.

When LDL is oxidized by free radicals, white blood cells in artery linings start attracting excessive amounts of LDL. The oxidized LDL forms fatty streaks on the inner arterial walls, and these streaks become the foundation of atherosclerosis.

In the study, samples of blood from people with normal blood cholesterol levels were taken, and their LDL was oxidized in test tubes, either with or without vitamin C. Next, the amount of oxidized LDL absorbed by the white blood cells was measured. Compared with the non-vitamin C blood samples, the blood with vitamin C prevented the oxidation of LDL, cutting its absorption by 93 percent. In a similar experiment, vitamin E blocked absorption of LDL by 45 percent. As antioxidants, vitamins C and E appear to neutralize free radicals, as this study suggests.[9]

Evidence is building that vitamin C has an anti-cancer effect as well – particularly against such cancers as those of the colon, mouth, larynx, and lung.[10]

Vitamin C is found in tomatoes, citrus fruits, strawberries, green peppers, potatoes, and dark green vegetables.

Vitamin D

This fat-soluble vitamin assists in the formation and maintenance of bones and teeth, is vital for a healthy nervous system, and helps protect the health of the heart. You cannot talk about vitamin D without mentioning calcium and phosphorus – two minerals that must be maintained in a constant ratio in the blood to be properly used by the body. Vitamin D helps maintain this ratio in the blood. Without vitamin D, calcium cannot be properly absorbed from food.

Most of your vitamin D requirements can be met by exposure to sunlight and by eating such foods as skim milk, tuna, and salmon.

Vitamin E

Vitamin E continues to show promise as an antioxidant, that special class of nutrients that fights free radicals. Animal studies have demonstrated that vitamin E helps protect white blood cells from this damage. Not only that, vitamin E appears to enhance the ability of white blood cells to destroy disease-causing bacteria.

Now there is evidence that vitamin E may have the same immune system-bolstering effects on humans that it does on animals. In a study at the USDA Human Research Center on Aging at Tufts University, a group of elderly people (age 60 and older) took 800 IUs of vitamin E a day, and another group took a placebo. The analysis of blood samples of the vitamin E group showed high levels of certain biochemicals that fight disease. In addition, the subjects' T-cells (cells that help other cells destroy invading agents) were secreting more interleukin-2, a bio-chemical that helps T-cells multiply. The analysis of the placebo group did not show the same results.[11]

A side effect of being active is that slight muscle cell damage can occur with vigorous exercise. As you jog, run, or cycle, you take in more oxygen than normal, thus exposing your muscle tissue to more of this highly reactive gas as well as to pollutants in the air. Taken together, oxygen and pollutants can upset the delicate chemical structure of the cell – a reaction known as "oxidative damage." Vitamin E's role is to help prevent this damage, and new research indicates that it may counter the effects of exercise-induced cell damage.[12]

In one study, these effects were observed in mountain climbers, whose intense, high altitude exercise is known to cause changes in blood levels, indicating damage to blood cells. One group was given 400 mg of vitamin E a day, while another group received a placebo. Both groups continued their intense climbs during the study. Tests showed that the supplemented climbers had less damage to red blood cells than did the placebo group.[13]

Vitamin E occurs naturally in vegetable oils, whole grain cereals, dried beans, and green, leafy vegetables – yet the content is not high. Consequently, many researchers feel that vitamin E supplements are more effective than foods as a means of getting adequate vitamin E.

If you decide to take vitamin supplements, take them with your meals. But remember: Do not take vitamin supplements without first consulting your physician. Anyone with high blood pressure should start with small amounts of vitamin E and increase gradually.

❧ *Key Points*

• Vitamins have specific metabolic roles to play in the body, yet no vitamin acts alone. All vitamins must be present in the correct balance to maintain good health.

• Nutritional supplementation is probably warranted – for several reasons. These include: low nutrient content of many foods as a result of soil depletion; poor bioavailability of many vitamins and minerals; nutrient depletion in food due to cooking; nutrition depletion due to exercise and stress; and dietary deficiencies.

• Research shows that most of the population does not eat nutritiously enough to meet the Recommended Daily Allowances (RDA).

• Vitamin A and beta carotene appear to have a protective effect against some forms of cancer.

• B-complex vitamins are involved in nearly every reaction that occurs in the body.

• New research on vitamin C shows that this nutrient may be a potent cholesterol fighter.

• Vitamin D assists in the formation of bones and teeth, is vital for the health of your nervous system, and helps protect the health of your heart.

• Vitamin E is a promising antioxidant, with a bolstering effect on the immune system.

8

❠ *Minerals and Other Amazing Nutrients*

MINERALS ARE IMPORTANT for the formation of body structures such as bones and tissue and are involved in many physiological processes, including metabolism and energy production. Referred to as "electrolytes," certain minerals are responsible for maintaining the fluid balance of the body. Sodium, calcium, and chloride are the main electrolytes in the fluid outside cells; potassium, magnesium, and phosphorus are found inside cellular fluid. Electrolytes provide a life-sustaining environment for cells and must be kept in constant balance for good health. Low levels of minerals and electrolytes can result in fatigue and other ill effects. These nutrients are lost through perspiration, so active people often have higher requirements.

Like vitamins, a mineral supplement should always be taken with meals – and only after consulting your physician.

Calcium

Of all minerals in the body, calcium is the most abundant. About 99 percent of the calcium in your body is deposited in bones and teeth. These structures are hardened and strengthened by calcium, working in combination with the mineral phosphorus. The remaining 1 percent of the body's calcium is concentrated in the soft tissues where it plays an essential role in muscle contraction, nerve transmission, blood coagulation, and the activity of the heart.

Dairy products are the best known of the calcium-rich foods, with a cup of skim milk supplying about 290 mg. Vegetables are high in calcium as well, and some of the best sources are kale, turnip greens, and broccoli. Another excellent source is canned salmon with bones.

Despite the abundance of calcium-rich foods, the bioavailability of calcium from food is low. In fact, only about 20 to 30 percent of the calcium you get from foods is absorbed. Certain foods and substances can interfere with the bioavailability of calcium. Whole grains are one example. The fiber in these foods tends to bind with calcium and carry it out of the body, causing depletion. Phytates (phosphorus groups) in fiber also block calcium absorption. The same is true of oxalic acid, a substance found in spinach, beet greens, and chard. (Phytates and oxalic acid do not block calcium absorption from other foods, however.) Certain factors can improve the absorption of calcium, especially the presence of vitamins A, C, D, and adequate dietary fat.[1]

The most well-known calcium deficiency is osteoporosis, which afflicts postmenopausal women. In this condition, bone mineral (calcium and phosphorus) is gradually lost from the inner cavity of the bone, weakening it and increasing susceptibility to bone fractures.

Both calcium supplementation and exercise increase bone mass in women. In a study using three groups of women over age 80, one group took a 750 mg calcium tablet every day. Another group exercised 30 minutes a day, three times a week. And a control group did neither of these but continued regular activities.

After three years, the control group had lost bone mass, while the other groups had gained bone mass. The group that exercised rebuilt the most bone – about 5.5 percent more than the control group.[2]

Another study of younger women aged 25 to 34 years old showed that a combination of regular exercise (running and walking) and high calcium intake – either by diet or supplementation – can build bone mass in the lumbar spine by up to 15 percent. The results suggest that calcium and exercise offer protection against osteoporosis in later years.[3]

Magnesium

Nutritionists have long known that the typical American diet is low in magnesium, a mineral that is involved in many metabolic functions. Increasingly, magnesium is becoming known as the "heart mineral" because of its protective effect on the heart. Research suggests that magnesium may be helpful in preventing angina (attacks of chest pain), lessening the damage of heart tissue in the aftermath of a heart attack, and treating patients with irregular heartbeats.[4]

Other research indicates that people who drink softened water (which is low in magnesium and calcium) have a higher incidence of heart attack and stroke than those who drink mineral-rich hard water.[5]

Here is something else to consider: Studies of magnesium levels in the blood suggest the possibility that a low-magnesium diet might actually draw magnesium from the body's soft tissues, such as the heart. Because magnesium is essential in maintaining healthy, smooth muscle cells, this "robbing effect" could damage the heart muscle.

Magnesium-rich foods include chick peas, beet greens, and turnip greens. If you decide to take a mineral supplement, make sure that the magnesium content is equal to or at least 70 percent of the calcium. Calcium cannot be metabolized without magnesium.

Potassium

Potassium serves the body in many ways. It assists the nerves in sending messages, helps digestive enzymes do their work, ensures proper muscle functioning (including that of the heart), and releases energy from protein, carbohydrates, and fats.

Potassium is one of the electrolytes that works with sodium in a sort of tug-of-war to regulate the distribution of fluids on either side of cell walls. Sodium is found in the fluids outside cells; potassium is inside cellular fluids. High sodium intake causes potassium to be drained from cells, while excess potassium drives sodium out. It is vital to health that the sodium and potassium be kept in natural equilibrium. A potassium deficiency, for example, can lead to irregular heart beats, muscular weakness, fatigue, and kidney and lung problems. Menus on the Lean Bodies program provide a potassium/sodium ratio of at least 2-to-1. This ratio is effective for maintaining the proper balance of these two minerals.

Runners who train and compete in hot weather have increased needs for potassium. This is because both heat and perspiration cause potassium losses. Use of diuretics or laxatives can also cause potassium depletion.

Some of the best sources of potassium are potatoes, lima beans, flounder, winter squash, spinach, and carrots. Food processing, however, tends to destroy the potassium content of foods. Being water soluble, potassium can be lost by cooking vegetables in water. That is why it is a good idea to steam vegetables or eat them raw.

Iron

This mineral helps create hemoglobin, a protein in your red blood cells that ferries oxygen from the lungs to the rest of your body. About 73 percent of the iron in your body is found in hemoglobin. If you have an iron deficiency (anemia), not enough hemoglobin is manufactured, and the supply of oxygen to body tissues is reduced. As the saying goes, you have "iron-poor blood" and feel rundown as a result.

There is more to the iron story than just its role in the blood, however. Iron deficiency affects brain function, endurance levels, and the immune system. It is one of the most common health problems in the world today.

In a study conducted by researchers at Massachusetts Institute of Technology, preschoolers who were mildly iron deficient had lower scores on behavioral tests than those children whose iron status was normal. The scores of the iron-deficient children significantly improved after about three months of iron therapy. Many other studies have found similar associations. Researchers, however, have not yet identified precisely how iron affects brain function, although it is believed that iron is important to the development and function of certain neurons.[6]

An iron deficiency can slow you down not only mentally but physically as well. Case in point: Researchers at the University of California studied the physical work capacity of 75 women, some of whom had severe iron deficiencies. The study found that the women with the lowest levels of iron stayed on the treadmill an average of eight minutes less than the others in the study. Furthermore, the iron-deficient women had twice as much lactate in their systems. Lactate is a chemical in the muscles that is associated with fatigue.[7] Additionally, studies of workers in developing countries have consistently found links between low iron levels in workers and reduced work capacity.

Iron is an important regulator of the immune system in both humans and animals. A low level of iron impairs the ability of lymphocytes (white blood cells in the lymphatic system) and phagocytes (white blood cells that fight bacterial invasion) to do their jobs. In short, an iron deficiency makes the immune system more vulnerable to attack from invading agents.[8]

Iron comes from two dietary sources: plants (nonheme iron) and animal protein (heme iron). Nonheme iron, however, is not well absorbed. Take spinach, for example. Even though this vegetable is rich in iron, only 1.4 percent of the mineral from spinach can be used by the body. To get enough iron from spinach, you would have to eat about three pounds of it of a day. In contrast, as much as 20 percent of iron from chicken, in the form of heme iron, is retained.[9]

You can improve your absorption of iron by combining foods in the manner explained in the Lean Bodies program. A meal combining chicken (a lean protein), spinach (a lean, fibrous vegetable), and a potato (a starchy carbohydrate) provides excellent sources of both heme and nonheme iron. In such a combination, the heme iron actually improves the absorption of the nonheme iron, and the high vitamin C content of the potato enhances the absorption of nonheme iron. The amino acids in the protein help escort iron into the system, and Vitamin C assists in changing the nonheme iron into a more useable form.

Boron

Found in tomatoes, green peppers, and other vegetables, this trace mineral has great importance in nutrition, especially in mineral metabolism. In a study of postmenopausal women, for example, boron supplementation greatly reduced the amount of calcium and magnesium excretion and increased blood levels of a natural form of estrogen. (Estrogen administration is the only known treatment that effectively slows the loss of calcium from bone in postmenopausal women.) The findings suggest that boron may be important in the prevention and treatment of osteoporosis.[10]

Chromium

Chromium is a mineral that helps turn carbohydrates into energy and plays a key role in stabilizing blood sugar. Nine out of 10 Americans are deficient in this nutrient, and the main reason is that the body cannot effectively absorb dietary sources of chromium – even though it is abundant in broccoli, potatoes, and other vegetables. Another problem is that diets high in simple sugars such as glucose and fructose rob the body of chromium, whereas diets rich in starchy carbohydrates preserve it.

In 1971, Dr. Arnold Schaffer, who was then head of the Food and Vitamin Division of the FDA, noted a correlation between low levels of chromium in the American diet and a rise in the incidence of diabetes. At the time, he stated that if chromium were increased in the average diet, he would expect to see a 50-percent reduction in diabetes in the population. New research now shows that chromium supplementation may indeed help lessen and even reverse the symptoms of diabetes, particularly type II diabetics. (Individuals with type II diabetes produce enough insulin but cannot process blood sugar properly.)

A 14-week study at Georgetown University in Washington, D.C., suggests that chromium supplementation may improve glucose tolerance – the ability to transport blood glucose into cells for use by the body. Chromium's effects were tested by giving supplemental chromium to 17 men and women, eight of whom had mild glucose intolerance, a pre-diabetic condition.

During the first four weeks of the study, all the participants ate a low-chromium diet. The participants were then divided into two groups. One group stayed on the diet but was given daily chromium supplements of 200 micrograms. The other group also continued to eat the low-chromium diet but took placebo pills instead of the supplements. Five weeks later, the diet/supplement regimen of the groups was reversed.

To measure the effects of chromium supplementation, the participants drank a sugary liquid. Blood sugar levels were then measured. In seven of the eight glucose-intolerant patients, blood sugar rose 50 percent less with chromium supplementation. As this study suggests, chromium supplementation may be a way to help reverse glucose intolerance.[11]

Where diabetes is concerned, chromium also works hand in hand with diet – one that is high in protein and complex carbohydrates. Protein is particularly important because it strengthens the function of the pancreas, which releases insulin. Also needed is the amino acid glycine, which converts to glucose in the body, and vitamin B_6, which has been found to prevent the build-up of dangerous plaque in the arteries – often a complication of diabetes.

Several diabetics enrolled in the Lean Bodies program have experienced remarkable improvements in their condition. Viv D., for example, is an insulin-dependent diabetic whose insulin requirements had been gradually increasing over the years. When I met him, he needed three injections a day, with 30 units of insulin per shot. After six weeks of following the program, he was able to reduce his insulin requirements by about one-third. In addition, he lost 10 pounds and has a better sense of well-being. Viv says that as he continues to shed pounds, his need for insulin will be reduced even more.

(Diabetics should always consult their physicians in matters regarding medication adjustments.)

Manganese

One of the trace minerals, manganese is involved in the formation of bone and cartilage. It also plays a role in protein, carbohydrate, and fat production. Deficiency symptoms include poor muscular coordination, abnormal brain function, glucose tolerance problems, and poor skeletal and cartilage formation. One cause of manganese deficiency appears to be the consumption of simple sugars. In one study of men and women, sugar was substituted for complex carbohydrates in a diet that provided ample dietary manganese. This substitution, however, caused manganese levels to drop.[12]

Low levels of manganese have been linked to osteoporosis. In one study, concentrations of serum manganese in osteoporotic women were found to be just 25 percent of the concentrations normally found in women.[13] This suggests that manganese may be an important mineral for women who are susceptible to osteoporosis because of the role it plays in bone formation.

Selenium

Selenium is a trace mineral that works together with vitamin E in affecting growth and metabolic functions. This mineral has become best known as an antioxidant because it preserves the elasticity of the skin. It has also been shown in research to have a protective effect against cancer.

Selenium is found in the bran of cereals, in tuna, and in such vegetables as broccoli and onions.

Zinc

Zinc does many things in the body. For example, it helps: absorb vitamins; break down carbohydrates; synthesize nucleic acid, which directs the manufacture of protein in cells; and regulate the growth and development of reproductive organs. Zinc is a component of the hormone insulin. Also, zinc is one of the trace minerals, along with boron, that appears to be a factor in preventing osteoporosis.

Elderly people may be at risk for zinc deficiencies, and this can affect immune function. This possibility was investigated in 173 elderly people in Florida, who were given a zinc supplement for four weeks. Their immune response improved significantly, leading the researchers to suggest that a zinc deficiency may cause immune disorders in the aged.[14]

Diets high in protein and whole grain products are usually high in zinc.

Lipotropics

Certain supplemental nutrients assist the body in the mobilization and metabolism of fat. These nutrients are called "lipotropics." If used as part of a supplement program, they should be taken with meals. A good formulation should contain all or most of the following:

Biotin. A B-complex vitamin, biotin assists in the oxidation of fatty acids and carbohydrates. Without it, the body cannot adequately metabolize fat.

Choline. This B-complex vitamin is a "first string" player among lipotropics. Its most vital function is regulating the amount of fat that accumulates in the liver, which is the body's first storage site for excess fat.

Another benefit of choline is that it helps emulsify cholesterol, preventing it from building up in the artery walls or gall bladder. Also, choline works to rid the body of toxins, poisons, and any drug residues.

Deficiencies in choline contribute to high blood pressure, hardening of the arteries, cirrhosis of the liver, lack of appetite, and retarded growth in children. Interestingly, hens will not lay eggs if they are deficient in choline.

Inositol. Closely associated with biotin and choline is the B-complex vitamin inositol. This nutrient stimulates the body's production of lecithin, a lipid-based component in the body that transports fats from the liver to the cells. Inositol is thus an important regulator of fat metabolism. It also helps reduce cholesterol by preventing the fatty deposits in the arteries that lead to atherosclerosis.

L-carnitine. Another important lipotropic is L-carnitine, a protein-like nutrient made by the body but also found in foods. Its main function is to assist the body in burning fat. In studies, L-carnitine appears to emulsify fat buildup in the arteries and internal organs. L-carnitine also stimulates the adrenal gland, which aids the body in using its fat reserves as fuel.

Betaine. This nutrient is a substance from which choline is formed and has similar functions.

Coenzyme Q10 (CoQ10)

One of the most widely prescribed drugs for cardiac disease and disease prevention in Japan is available in the United States, not by prescription, but as a nutritional supplement. That nutrient is Coenzyme Q10 (abbreviated as CoQ10) and is technically known as ubiquinone. This substance is also found naturally inside the mitochondria of the cell, where it is involved in the conversion of food to energy. Supplementally, it is a nutrient that appears to have many health-giving properties. For example, it helps improve cardiac function, strengthens the immune system, and may enhance the quality of overall health. Many studies have been done supporting CoQ10's benefits as an oral supplement.

One study, conducted in Japan and published in *The New England Journal of Medicine*, demonstrates CoQ10's promise as an antioxidant in fighting cholesterol. Researchers measured the ratios of plasma ubiquinone levels to plasma LDL cholesterol levels in two groups – 245 healthy individuals (186 men and 59 women) and 72 patients (38 men and 34 women) who had ischemic heart disease or early signs of it. LDL cholesterol, the study pointed out, can accumulate in the arterial walls and, when oxidized, may cause hardening of the arteries.

In the patient group, the levels of ubiquinone were lower and the levels of LDL cholesterol were higher than in the normal subjects. These findings led the researchers to suggest that the ratio of LDL cholesterol to ubiquinone may be an indicator of the risk for developing atherosclerosis and that ubiquinone itself may help in the prevention of this disease.[15]

Appearing as a guest with me on the "Weekend Workout" on KLIF in Dallas was Luke Bucci, Ph.D., a noted clinical nutritionist who has conducted human research studies on CoQ10. He related a study from the University of Texas in Austin that found that AIDS patients have very low levels of CoQ10 in their blood. As part of this study, the patients were given very large doses of the supplement to boost blood levels back to normal. In conjunction with regular medical treatment, the patients' symptoms were reduced. The findings suggest that CoQ10 may have merit in fighting immune system disorders.[16]

If you are interested in supplementing your diet with CoQ10, how much should you take? Dr. Bucci recommends 30 mg a day if you are moderately active, and between 60 mg and 100 mg if you are more active and participate in weight training or endurance sports.

Garlic

This centuries-old remedy may have preventive and curative properties in a wide range of ailments, including heart disease, cancer, immune system disorders, among others. Garlic, it seems, contains more than 200 biologically active compounds that appear to positively alter the course of many illnesses.

For example, garlic supplements have been shown to lower LDL cholesterol, a major risk factor for heart disease. In a study conducted by B. Lau, a leading scientist in this area, four capsules of a garlic preparation (Kyolic Aged Garlic Extract) were given daily to people with high cholesterol. A control group received a placebo.

In the group taking garlic, levels of cholesterol in the blood dropped significantly, while those of the control group showed no change. LDL cholesterol, in particular, decreased in the garlic group, and HDL, which protects against the build-up of arterial plaque, increased. Many other studies on garlic preparations have reported similar findings.[17]

Other research has shown that supplemental garlic enhances immune function, provides antioxidant effects, helps the body dissolve blood clots, and may prevent the formation of carcinogens that form in the stomach. Believe it or not, there is an enormous amount of energy being channeled into the study of garlic. In fact, I have mounds of research studies on garlic on my desk to prove it!

! *Key Points*

- Minerals are involved in the formation of body structures and in metabolism and energy production.
- Calcium is the most abundant mineral in the body and
plays an essential role in building bones and teeth. A calcium deficiency can contribute to osteoporosis.
- Boron and manganese are important trace minerals
that appear to play a role in the prevention of osteoporosis.
- Magnesium has a protective effect on the heart.
- Potassium is important because of the role it plays in
metabolism and the regulation of body fluids.
- Iron is involved in oxygen transport, brain function,
endurance levels, and the immune system. Iron deficiency
is one of the most common medical problems in the world
today.
- Chromium is a a trace mineral that helps stabilize
blood sugar. Nine out of 10 Americans are deficient in this
nutrient, primarily because of its poor availability. Chromium supplementation appears to be helpful in lessening
the symptoms of type II diabetes.
- Selenium is a well-known antioxidant that shows promise in fighting cancer.
- Zinc is a trace mineral involved in a number of functions in the body, including metabolism, the synthesis of
nucleic acid, and the development of reproductive organs.
- Lipotropics are a class of nutrients that assist the body
in the metabolism and mobilization of fats.

• Widely prescribed in Japan for heart disease, CoQ10 is available in the United States as a nutritional supplement. Research shows that CoQ10 helps improve cardiac function, reduce cholesterol, and strengthen the immune system.

• A centuries-old remedy, garlic shows promise in treating heart disease, cancer, and immune system disorders.

9

✶ *Fat-Burning/*
Health-Building Exercise

THE TURNING POINT for attorney Harvey A., age 59, came during a treadmill test. Thirty pounds overweight and out of condition, Harvey could barely stay on the treadmill three minutes – not even long enough for his doctor to tell if anything was wrong with him. To make matters worse, Harvey was being outpaced at the next treadmill by a 75-year-old man, who turned in a performance of 12 minutes.

"The experience depressed me," Harvey recalls. "I was walking like a very old man."

Determined to make some changes, Harvey started the Lean Bodies program. Along with it, he began a walking program, with an initial workout of just 20 minutes of slow walking a few times a week. Six months later, he was walking four miles a day, six times a week. He lost 40 pounds and dropped his total cholesterol from 323 to 191. In addition, Harvey's doctor took him off blood pressure medication.

As it does with many people, the bodyfat crept up on Bill A. By the time he was 61, Bill weighed 330 pounds, with a bodyfat percentage of 56. "I was very short of breath and unable to walk up even the slightest grade. I didn't have any ambition about anything. So I decided to do something about my condition."

Bill began the Lean Bodies program, and early on realized that exercise could maximize his progress. "Because the program recommends weight training, I decided to get a personal trainer. Next to changing my eating habits, that was the best thing I did."

Bill's workout regimen is impressive. He trains at a gym three times a week with weights. Before weight training, he complained of aches and pains from head to toe. "Not anymore. I used to blame the pain on age but now I realize it was just being out of shape. My body feels so much stronger today."

In addition to weight training, Bill works out aerobically three times a week, either walking or riding his stationary bicycle. "I've reached the point now where I'd like to start jogging," he says.

Of course, the best news of all is that Bill has dropped 50 pounds of bodyfat and is still losing.

The Exercise Connection

It is no secret that exercise is a critical component of any bodyfat loss program. In my Lean Bodies classes, I encourage my clients to pursue two kinds of exercise – aerobic exercise and weight training. Each is vital for fitness and peak health.

Aerobic exercise such as walking, jogging, or bicycling is the only type of physical activity that directly burns bodyfat. For fat to be burned, oxygen must be present, and this occurs through aerobic exercise. At the start of the exercise, your body uses carbohydrates, stored as glycogen in the muscles, for energy. Then, the energy source changes from carbohydrates to fat. After about 20 minutes of working out, fat is released from cells in the form of fatty acids to be used as energy. Aerobic exercise boosts your uptake of oxygen, and this trains your muscles to burn fat as fuel.

In addition, aerobic exercise strengthens your heart muscle, raises the level of high-density lipoprotein (HDL) cholesterol (called the "good kind" because it helps prevent clogged arteries), and lowers your blood pressure. These all help reduce your chances of heart attack and stroke.

When exercising aerobically, you should try to work up to a heart rate of between 130 and 150 beats a minute, depending on your age. This is your target heart rate (THR), and reaching it puts your body into a fat-burning mode.

To determine your individual rate, take the number 220, subtract your age, and then multiply that number by 75 percent. Learn to take your pulse by placing your fingers over the carotid artery located on either side of your neck. Count the number of beats that occur during a 10-second period. Multiply that number by 6 to arrive at your pulse rate per minute. If you are at your target heart rate, you are burning fat.

An indirect way to burn fat is by weight training. This is the application of resistance (dumbbells, barbells, or special weight training machines) against muscles. Resistance actually breaks down muscle fibers. The repair of these fibers is part of what makes muscles get larger and stronger.

The more muscle you have, the better your body can burn fat. This is because muscle is the body's most metabolically active tissue. For every new pound of muscle you put on with exercise, you use about 50 to 100 calories more a day.

If you are like many people, you probably have a lot of misconceptions about weight training. Put all those misconceptions aside. Weight training (also called resistance training) tones, develops, and strengthens the muscles of the body and is one of the best activities you can adopt for health and longevity. Here is why:

The loss of muscle tone and strength is a process that begins in your late twenties – unless you undertake a regular exercise program that includes weight training. Weight training is the only exercise known to regenerate vital body tissue (muscle), regardless of age.

In a study at the Hebrew Rehabilitation Center for the Aged in Boston, six women and four men ranging in age from 86 to 96 were put on a monitored weight training program three times a week for eight weeks. Their exercises focused primarily on leg work.

At the end of the study, the subjects' strength had increased by an average of 174 percent, and total mid-thigh muscle area increased by 9 percent. The researchers concluded that muscle strength and development can be favorably altered by weight training.[1] It goes to show that no matter how old – or how young – you are, you can benefit from exercise.

There is a growing body of evidence that weight training has cardiovascular benefits, including improved blood cholesterol levels, increased efficiency in the way the heart does its job, and decreased blood pressure.

Combining weight training with aerobic exercise doubles the fat-burning effect, as Alan N. discovered. Alan, age 21, had battled a weight problem most of his life. On his last diet, he lost more than 50 pounds by living on fruit juice and yogurt. Soon afterward, though, he ballooned up to 250 pounds.

Alan's brother invited him to work in a gym he was opening, and Alan was excited about the opportunity. "But he hadn't seen me since I had gained all the weight," Alan recalls. "When I got off the plane, he was ready to shoot me."

The very next day, Alan started the Lean Bodies program, eating between five and seven meals a day. For aerobic exercise, he walked on a treadmill for a minimum of 45 minutes a day every day and started lifting weights three days a week. In just two months, Alan lost 40 pounds, and the loss continued. "Right now, I'm at 180 pounds, thanks to nutrition, aerobics, and weight training.

I've kept the weight off for almost two years. I've never had that experience before."

Health Benefits Of Exercise

Whether you do aerobic exercise, lift weights, or both, staying active leads to greater levels of physical and mental health. In addition to its fat-burning effect, exercise, when accompanied by proper nutrition, is proving to be an important preventive factor in many diseases, some of them life threatening. Here are some examples:

Arthritis

People with arthritis typically have either rheumatoid arthritis or osteoarthritis. With rheumatoid arthritis, there is inflammation in the synovial lining of the joints, leading to cartilage and bone damage. With osteoarthritis, cartilage in joints deteriorates, and the condition usually affects weight-bearing joints such as hips and knees. Joint pain, loss of motion, muscular weakness, and reduced mobility are the results of both types of arthritis.

Performed under the recommendation of a physician, aerobic exercise is proving to have many benefits for arthritic patients. In one study at the University of Michigan, 23 patients were divided into one of three aerobic exercise programs using stationary bicycles. Each group exercised at a different level of intensity, and a fourth group, serving as the control, did not exercise. The researchers observed that aerobic exercise improved aerobic capacity, enhanced endurance, and reduced the severity of painful joints.[2]

In addition to stationary bicycling, other forms of exercise have been found to be helpful for arthritic sufferers. These include swimming, pool exercises, walking, cross country ski machines, rowing, and low impact aerobic dancing.

Cancer

Only in the past several years has exercise been studied for its role in reducing the risk of cancer. A study published in 1985 in *The British Journal of Cancer* observed that athletic women had a significantly lower risk of developing cancers of the breast and reproductive system than did nonathletic women. [3]

Regular exercise also appears to lessen the risk of colon cancer. In a major study of Harvard alumni, researchers analyzed data from 17,148 participants to investigate the potential link between physical activity and the reduced risk of colon cancer. Alumni were asked about their exercise habits and sports activities. It turned out that those who were either highly active or moderately active had about half the risk of developing colon cancer as the inactive alumni.

The protective effect of physical activity may be related to the fact that exercise cuts the transit time of food through the intestines, providing less opportunity for carcinogens to interact with the lining of the colon, according to the researchers. [4]

Obesity is a risk factor for cancer, and studies over the past 50 years support this, according to the National Cancer Institute (NCI). Cancers of the uterus, gallbladder, breast, kidney, endometrium, and colon have all been linked to obesity. Because exercise, in conjunction with proper nutrition, fights obesity, it may serve as a protective factor against these cancers. [5]

Cholesterol

According to the American Heart Association, cardiovascular illness (diseases of the heart and blood vessels) kills approximately one American every 32 seconds. In a year, that adds up to more Americans than died in World Wars I and II and the Korean and Viet Nam wars. [6]

Medical experts believe that a sizable share of these deaths can be prevented if people take better care of themselves with good health habits such as proper nutrition, not smoking, and exercise.

Major culprits in the development of cardiovascular disease are fatty substances called cholesterol and triglycerides. Cholesterol is made by the body and required for many vital functions, and triglycerides are fats that travel in the blood and are eventually stored in fat cells. When too much of these fatty substances travels in the bloodstream, the excess gradually finds its way to the inner arterial walls, where it is deposited, eventually obstructing the arteries.

Exercise favorably alters the lipoprotein profile so that high-density lipoproteins (HDL) are raised while low-density lipoproteins (LDL) are lowered. This effect has been repeatedly shown in research.

The cardiovascular benefits of vigorous walking, for example, were demonstrated in a study of 31 healthy, sedentary women (age 61 to 81) who walked three times a week for eight weeks. By the end of the eight-week period, the women's triglycerides and LDL cholesterol had dropped significantly, while HDL cholesterol had increased. As the researchers pointed out, "This study provides evidence that sedentary older women who choose exercise as a means of altering a less than optimal lipid profile can effect modest changes in serum lipids and lipoproteins in a relatively short time."[7]

Weight training produces similar effects. In one study, 11 untrained men (age 40 to 55) exercised for 16 weeks on a weight training program using machines. When tested following the study, the men had cut their LDL cholesterol by 5 percent and upped their HDL cholesterol by 13 percent. The findings suggest that regular weight training may reduce risk factors for cardiovascular disease.[8, 9]

Diabetes

This sugar metabolism disorder is the third leading killer disease in the United States. Diabetics have an excess of glucose (blood sugar) circulating in their bodies. Normally, glucose is taken up by the cells to be used for energy – a process that requires the hormone insulin. Insulin signals the receptors on the outer cell membrane, allowing the cell to open up so that glucose can enter.

In type I diabetics, not enough insulin is produced, and consequently, muscle, fat, and liver cells cannot absorb glucose, which is needed for energy. These patients, who typically get the disease at a young age, must therefore depend on daily injections of the hormone to survive.

Most diabetics are type II, a form that usually shows up after age 40 in people who are overweight and not physically active and in those with a family history of diabetes. In type II diabetics, insulin is produced but the cells are not sensitive to it, probably because there are fewer insulin receptors on the outer cell walls. Glucose, therefore, has trouble entering cells. Type II diabetes is easier to manage than type I and does not require insulin injections.

All diabetics are at risk for a host of complications, including obesity, eye problems, nerve damage, kidney disease, and cardiovascular disease. Cardiovascular disease, in fact, is the leading cause of death among diabetics.

In addition to proper diet and insulin (for type I diabetics), exercise plays a key role in the management of this disease. Type II diabetes is thought to be a lifestyle disease linked to sedentary habits and poor diet. In fact, new research is offering proof that regular exercise may prevent type II diabetes.[10]

Exercise keeps blood sugar levels in normal range. The exact mechanism by which this occurs is unknown, although the theory is that exercise may increase the insulin receptors on cell walls or cause cellular changes that let glucose get inside cells. Second, exercise lowers total cholesterol and improves the ratio of HDL cholesterol to LDL cholesterol, thereby reducing the threat of cardiovascular disease.

Diabetic patients who begin exercise programs are advised to self-monitor glucose levels before and after exercise. This is because exercise causes changes in blood sugar levels, and these changes must be closely tracked so that the proper adjustments in insulin and/or diet can be made.

Emotional Health

From running to weight training, exercise is a powerful remedy against many emotional problems of daily living. The mood-lifting benefits of exercise have important application in clinical circles – especially because mental disorders have become a major public health problem.

Depression alone affects one out of every four Americans, according to the President's Commission of Mental Health. It is an emotional disorder with a wide range of symptoms, including withdrawal, inactivity, loss of appetite, feelings of helplessness, and anxiety. In addition to the many therapies available, exercise is emerging as an important adjunct to treatment.

In one study, 30 to 40 minutes of walking and running three times a week compared favorably with psychotherapy in the treatment of eight depressed patients. Six of the patients were diagnosed as "essentially well" after three weeks of exercise therapy, and they stayed that way for one year afterwards.[11]

Another study examined the responses of 43 depressed women to either aerobic exercise (dancing, jogging, and running), relaxation exercises, and non-exercise. The women who exercised aerobically experienced significantly greater decreases in depression than did all the other participants. The researchers concluded that "participation in a program of strenuous aerobic exercise was effective for reducing depression."[12]

Exercise has also been connected with enhanced self-esteem. A study at Auburn University found that male students who weight-trained for 16 weeks showed significantly more improvement in self-esteem than a control group who listened to health lectures during the same period.[13] Similar findings have been reported in studies of women who work out with weights.

Hypertension (High Blood Pressure)

Known as the silent killer, hypertension afflicts about 60 million Americans, half of whom do not know they have it. Hypertension is a serious condition because it contributes to heart attacks and strokes. Blood pressure exceeding 140/90 spells danger and should be brought under control.

Many studies have shown that regular exercise lowers blood pressure by maintaining the health of the circulatory system. Yet exercise is only one part of the prescription for hypertension; others include restricting salt intake, cutting down on alcohol and caffeine, quitting smoking, losing bodyfat, and taking blood pressure medication.

Many people on the Lean Bodies program have been able to lower their blood pressure by following the food plan and exercising regularly. Gene S., age 60, had dangerously high blood pressure when he began the program. He started exercising every morning and eating all the recommended foods. Eventually, his blood pressure dropped to a healthy range. Plus, he lost 15 pounds.

Osteoporosis

As you get older, your bones lose vital minerals, mainly bone-building calcium. This can result in osteoporosis. In men, the loss of minerals can begin at about age 50, but in women it can start as early as ages 30 to 35. By age 70, some women may lose up to 70 percent of their bone mineral mass. Although the exact cause of this demineralization has not been pinpointed, contributing factors include hormonal changes, nutritional deficiencies, and inactivity. Prevention and treatment of osteoporosis typically focus on nutrition, calcium and trace mineral supplementation, hormonal medication, and exercise.

Exercise appears to prevent a significant portion of bone mineral loss associated with aging. Exercise stimulates bone growth, leading to greater mineral content and thicker bones. Studies of athletes provide the best proof of this effect. Weight lifters, throwers, runners, soccer players, and ballet dancers are among the categories of athletes who have strong, dense bones.[14]

Recent research indicates that the best type of exercise for preventing osteoporosis appears to be weight training. A study at the University of Arizona looked at groups of 40 women, ages 17 to 38. Some were bodybuilders; others were competitive runners; and still others were swimmers and recreational runners. For comparison, a control group was made up of women who did not exercise. When measured, the average bone mineral content of the bodybuilders was consistently greater than that of the runners, swimmers, and controls.[15]

Premenstrual Tension

Premenstrual tension (PMS) is a combination of physical and emotional symptoms that typically occur a week or two before menstruation. PMS appears to be caused by a number of factors, including water retention, hormonal imbalances, hypoglycemia, and vitamin B_6 deficiency.

Many researchers believe that exercise helps alleviate PMS symptoms. A study by Jerilynn C. Prior, M.D., University of British Columbia in Vancouver, showed that women who exercised aerobically for six months had less breast tenderness, fluid retention, and other symptoms – when compared to a control group that did not exercise. Dr. Prior believes that her findings are related to higher levels of endorphins released through exercise.[16] Endorphins are a group of proteins in the body that have analgesic properties.

Designing Your Exercise Plan

Whether it is fat loss, a better shape, heart health, or relief from stress you are after, the message is clear: Regular exercise is a vital element in improving the quality of your life and your health.

The first step in designing an exercise plan is to decide your reasons for working out. What are your exercise goals? For example, do you want to:

• Burn bodyfat?
• Build muscle?
• Tone specific body parts such as hips and thighs?
• Enhance cardiovascular conditioning?
• Prevent or manage disease?
• All of the above?

The answers to those questions (your goals) will help you select the type of exercise to pursue. But there are other factors to consider as well. Prior knee injuries, for example, would make jogging inadvisable. Some forms of exercise may simply be inconvenient for you to follow on a regular basis. Others may not appeal to you. After all, you are more likely to stick to your exercise program if you enjoy it.

It is a good idea to learn all you can about exercise. Lack of knowledge is one of the greatest obstacles to exercise, particularly on how to exercise. For example, one common misconception is that you have to work out very hard, often to the point of exhaustion, to get healthier. Not true! In fact, overexertion can tear down your body's resistance to disease.

Another misconception is that the results of exercise happen quickly, when in fact they occur only through consistent workouts over time. That is why you must begin to think of exercise as a lifetime commitment, not something you will do for a short time.

What follows are eight popular forms of aerobic exercise, with guidelines on how to begin each. Always consult your physician before starting an exercising program.

Aerobic Dance. This activity is by far the most popular form of aerobic exercise, with more than 23 million participants. Aerobic dance is a great fat-burner, it gives an excellent cardiovascular work-out, and it exercises all major muscle groups – not to mention that aerobic dance is also fun.

The safest form of aerobic dance is the low-impact variety, in which at least one foot remains on the floor during the aerobic part of the session. Unlike regular aerobic dance, there are no jumps; instead, the exercise uses large upper body movements and relies on kicks, high steps, lunges, and other wide range-of-motion moves. These actions lessen the stress on joints, making low-impact aerobics a safer alternative for most people than regular aerobic dance. In many low-impact aerobics classes, hand or ankle weights are added to the exercises to make them more demanding. Stepping up and down on small benches as part of the dance routine is popular too – and intense. And, a recent study showed that combining hand-held weights with bench stepping burned more calories than just bench stepping by itself.[17]

Before joining an aerobics class, make sure that the instructors have been certified by a reputable organization and are trained in CPR.

A convenient alternative to attending aerobic dance classes is using exercise videos. They are handy if you do not have a lot of time to spend going from home to class and back again. They are also a good idea if you are self-conscious about going to a health club.

There are drawbacks, however. These include lack of instructor feedback on form and technique, potential injury from working out alone, and lack of the camaraderie you get from an exercise class.

Bicycling. This is a great aerobic workout and one that also improves muscle tone in the legs. It is not all leg work though, because your upper body works hard to maintain balance. To strengthen your cardiovascular system, you must ride at speeds faster than 15 miles per hour. That is when you start matching the efficiency of running.

If you are new to biking, you should first get accustomed to the bike and learn the basics of riding. Start out by biking up to 20 minutes a day at a low to moderate speed. From there, gradually increase your time to 30 minutes at a steady pace. Add about five minutes a week (up to about 60 minutes) while increasing your speed to achieve your target heart rate.

A popular alternative to biking is stationary cycling. With most of these bikes, you can adjust the resistance to make the workout more intense. The computerized versions have programs that simulate hilly terrain and other challenging courses.

Some people find stationary cycling a bit boring. But if you do it while watching TV, reading a good book, or listening to music through headphones, your stint on the bike will zip by.

Cross Country Ski Machines. These are designed to simulate the cross country ski experience – one of the best aerobic conditioners around. At first, these machines take some getting used to. As you glide, you must shift your weight over the ball of the foot that is headed backward. Next, shift your weight onto the foot gliding forward. If you do not, you will just be shuffling your legs back and forth. Try not to watch your feet either so that you stay upright rather than hunched forward. Once you master the rhythm of the movement, use the arm mechanism for extra intensity.

Jogging/Running. If you have never exercised before, you might not give jogging a second thought. That is what researchers at the University of Nebraska discovered when they surveyed the attitudes of men and women toward regular jogging. Non-exercisers, according to the survey, thought jogging required too much discipline and too much time. Plus, they felt jogging would wear them out.[18]

Many people who start our program are nonexercisers with some of the same preconceived notions. Ruth B. is a good example. About to turn 40, Ruth entered the program to lose bodyfat. "I didn't want to be fat at 40," she says.

When I suggested that she start jogging to speed up the fat-burning process, at first she laughed. But within a month, she took my advice, jogging at a slow pace for about 20 minutes each time. Today, she jogs four miles a day. "Jogging is so easy now that it feels like walking," Ruth says. Also, she lost the bodyfat she wanted to shed, and her total cholesterol dropped by 52 points.

Jogging and running are excellent ways to burn fat and achieve cardiovascular fitness, if done consistently. Generally speaking, the difference between jogging and running has to do with speed. If you are moving less than six miles an hour, you are jogging; faster than that, you are running.

As with any form of exercise, proper form is essential. To jog or run properly, you should maintain an upright position, with your head up. Hold your arms slightly away from your body, and bend your elbows so that your forearms are parallel to the ground. It is best to hit the ground with your heel first, rocking your foot forward and then pushing off the ball of your foot. As you jog or run, simply breathe normally.

To start your jogging or running program, set an initial goal of one mile, and gradually try to work up to achieving it. Increase your goal as distances are met. Depending on your level of conditioning, jog or run three times a week for a minimum of 30 minutes each time. As your fitness improves, so will your distances and times.

Stair Climbing Machines. Introduced in the 1980s, these machines are now a fixture in many health clubs and home gyms. The motorized versions feature computerized readouts of such information as the number of calories burned and flights climbed. An advantage of stair climbing machines is that they work large muscle groups in the back, buttocks, and legs, and this gives you a harder, more intense workout. This is in contrast to stationary bicycles which primarily work the quadriceps of the frontal thigh.

These machines work against your weight as you pump the foot pedals, one after the other. Various programs of intensity can be selected, according to your level of conditioning. Avoid leaning on the handrails as you pump. By leaning, you place too much stress on your shoulders and back and limit the aerobic intensity of the exercise.

Before exercising on a stair climbing machine, it is a good idea to stretch your legs to minimize the possibility of injury. Also, watch your footing as you pump the pedals in order to maintain your balance. Stair climbing causes a rapid rise in blood pressure, so people with hypertension should be extremely cautious.

Swimming. This activity is a very beneficial form of exercise because it strengthens both the cardiovascular system and all large muscle groups. Much of the muscular work involved is on the upper body, particularly the shoulders. Your body is buoyant in water, and this prevents potential strain.

Unlike many other types of exercise, swimming requires prior skill and mastery of strokes, including the crawl, breast stroke, side stroke, and backstroke. If you decide to swim for fitness, start with 30 minutes of swimming three times a week. To realize the aerobic and conditioning benefits from swimming, you must swim at a pace, intensity, and duration that challenge your heart rate, lungs, and muscles. As with any aerobic exercise, swimming has to be vigorous enough to elevate your heart rate to your target and keep it there for at least 20 minutes.

Treadmills. Up until recently, treadmills were used almost exclusively by competitive runners and cardiovascular physicians. Today, however, these devices have become popular workout tools for the masses, not only in gyms but in homes as well.

In addition to giving you a great aerobic workout, treadmills work the legs and buttocks. The motorized versions let you set the challenge by adjusting the speed of the moving belt, the elevation of its grade, or both. Some models feature digital displays that tell you how many calories you have burned and miles walked.

The non-motorized models are harder to use than their mechanized counterparts. The belt tends to drag, and you end up using energy on pushing rather than walking.

Before starting, step on the sides of the machine, not the belt. Once it begins moving, step on the belt carefully. For safety and balance, always hold the handrail. Walk at a pace that keeps up with the speed of the belt. To dismount, step on the sides of the machine again and then stop the machine by pushing the appropriate button.

Walking. If you have never exercised before, I suggest that you begin with a walking program. Walking is a natural movement that just about everyone can do, anywhere and anytime, weather permitting.

Like many of the people in our Lean Bodies classes, walking is the exercise of choice for Ronnie P., a restaurant executive. At five-foot-nine, Ronnie started the program weighing 205 pounds. Four to five mornings a week, he walks for 45 minutes on a hilly route and sprints 200 yards during his walk. His weight came off very fast. In three months, he lost 40 pounds. "Eating the right foods and exercising moderately – that's all it takes," he says. "You do not have to suffer or run hard – just enough to elevate your heart rate for about 25 minutes."

When walking, take normal strides but pump your arms in a swinging motion. This pumping action increases the aerobic benefits of walking. Your heel should hit first and then roll on to the ball of your foot.

It is important to walk briskly enough to attain your target heart rate. How fast is that? Data collected from a study at the University of Massachusetts provides a good rule of thumb. In the study, researchers tested men and women of various age groups to identify the minimum walking pace (in miles per hour) required to achieve their target heart rate. The results were as follows:[19]

Minimum Pace Required to Achieve THR

Men (30-39)	4.0 mph
Women (30-39)	3.5 mph
Men (40-49)	3.8 mph
Women (40-49)	3.5 mph

Men (50-59)   3.9 mph
Women (50-59)   2.9 mph

Men (60-69)   3.5 mph
Women (60-69)   3.0 mph

Try to increase your distance a little more each day. As you get in better shape, add hand-held weights to your walking program. By carrying hand weights (one to three pounds each) and swinging your arms vigorously as you walk, you can expend as much energy as you would with a slow jog.

If you are new to walking, begin the first week with short walks – about 15 minutes each. Increase your walks by about five minutes each week until you can walk 45 minutes or more each time. In the beginning, walk three times a week. As your conditioning improves, increase to four, five or more times a week.

A Closer Look At Weight Training

The reasons for adding weight training to your exercise routine are compelling: to reshape your body into more proportional contours, to get stronger, to increase lean mass as well as bone mass, and to strengthen the heart.

Weight training programs can be quite diverse. Some people work out four to six times a week, dividing the body up and working certain body parts on specific days. If you are new to weight training, however, your best bet is to work your entire body three days a week, on nonconsecutive days. This schedule gives your muscles time to rest so that they can respond by increasing in size and strength.

A good weight training routine for beginners consists of about three sets of 10 exercises using dumbbells, barbells or weight training machines. On the first set of each exercise, use a light weight and perform approximately 12 to 15 repetitions. Increase the poundage on the second set so that you can do about 10 to 12 repetitions. On the last set, up your poundage even more, using a weight that lets you lift about six to eight repetitions. By progressively increasing your weights from workout to workout, you challenge your muscles to develop, tone, and strengthen.

Here is a good starter routine for beginning weight trainers:

Monday / Wednesday / Friday

EXERCISE	BODY PART	REPS	SETS
Leg Extension	Thighs	15, 12, 10	3
Leg Curl	Hamstrings	15, 12, 10	3
Dumbbell Bench Press	Chest	15, 12, 10	3
Pulldowns	Back	15, 12, 10	3
Dumbbell Press	Shoulders	15, 12, 10	3
Arm Curl	Biceps	15, 12, 10	3
Triceps Pressdown	Triceps	15, 12, 10	3
Calf Raises	Calves	15, 12, 10	3
Abdominal Crunches	Abdominals	15, 12, 10	3

As you start lifting weights, first learn the correct exercise technique by working with a qualified instructor or trainer. For example:

1. To maximize body mechanics, you must maintain the proper position during your workout. Use strict form. Be careful to move

only the joints and body parts specified for each exercise.

2. Range of motion is the full path of an exercise, from extension to contraction and back again. To get the most from every repetition, lift the weight through a complete range of motion.

3. Stress muscle groups with maximum intensity. Always strive to progressively increase your poundages. That is the only way to insure optimal results.

4. Do not "overtrain." Some people get so hooked on weight training that they overdo it by working out too much. Each workout should be followed by a day of rest to let the muscles recuperate, strengthen, and grow.

5. Women should not be afraid of becoming "muscle-bound." The major reason men are capable of developing large muscles is the presence of the male hormone testosterone in their bodies. Women do not have this hormone and therefore cannot build as much muscle as men can.

Weight Training Safety

Unsafe weight training habits can result in injuries that are both painful and frustrating. After all, who wants to be put out of action by an injury? Fortunately, most injuries are preventable. All it takes is greater safety awareness while working out, at home or in a gym.

So the next time you are exercising, watch for unsafe conditions in your workout area and concentrate on correcting poor training habits. Here is what to look for:

Gym maintenance. Regular upkeep of equipment by gym owners is essential for safety. Items such as frayed cables, loosely mounted equipment, or broken machines should be fixed quickly or temporarily taken out of service until repairs can be made. Otherwise, the potential for serious injury remains.

Gym members are often the first to spot equipment problems. So it is a good idea to report these conditions immediately.

Plates, dumbbells, and other pieces of equipment that litter the floor create tripping hazards. That is why you should return equipment to its proper place after using it. Not only is this a safe practice, it is a courtesy to other weight trainers.

In addition, padding that is not regularly soaped down is a great breeding place for bacteria. So all equipment should be regularly cleaned and dusted, a responsibility of the gym owner or your responsibility if you have a home gym.

How to dress. Wear comfortable clothing that lets your skin breathe. Clothing that is too loose can snag on equipment. On the other hand, tight garb such as leotards made from synthetic fibers can lead to skin irritations.

Jewelry is a definite no-no in a gym. Not only is it inappropriate, it can easily catch on pulleys, handles, and other protruding objects. If you wear a wedding band, consider using weight lifting gloves. These help prevent calluses on your palms.

Using safety equipment. Barbells, dumbbells, and machines come with various safety features. Collars, for example, are fittings placed on the ends of free weight bars. They secure the plates to keep them from sliding off.

Certain benches have rails to catch the bar before it can trap you after a failed lift. Racks for performing exercises such as the squat let you easily load and unload the barbell after you have completed a set.

Machines are equipped with straps and seatbelts to keep your body properly aligned during exercises. They are also engineered to adjust to individual heights – a feature that is both a safety consideration and a design element to guarantee that the machine properly isolates the muscles.

Proper form. Proper technique can never be over-emphasized. With free weights, be sure to take a firm grip on the bar so you will not accidentally drop the weights. On standing exercises, distribute your weight equally on each leg. This will keep you from losing your balance and possibly injuring yourself. Also, bend your knees slightly to protect your lower back. No matter what the exercise, practice correct body alignment.

Gym "literacy." Do you understand how the equipment in your gym works? If not, take time to ask questions and get them answered. A thorough knowledge of how equipment is used can help keep you injury-free. And the more you know about the tools of weight training, the more successful you will be at getting in shape.

Using spotters. Another way to help ensure a safe workout (and a productive one) is to train with a "spotter," a responsible partner who understands proper lifting technique and safe exercise performance.

Although many weight trainers prefer to work out alone, certain exercises, such as squats, bench presses, and overhead shoulder presses, do require assistance. Lifters depend on spotters for their safety during these exercises.

A spotter lifts the bar off the rack and then guides it back to the rack after the completion of the set, and loads and unloads plates for you. Most importantly, your spotter encourages you and coaches you on correct form. When it is your turn to spot, you have the same responsibilities.

Know your limits. Handling weights that are too heavy can lead to strains, a condition characterized by swelling and pain in muscles, and pulls, which are acute tears of muscle fibers. To avoid these injuries, increase your poundages gradually. Do not overdo. Then give your muscles enough time to recover – at least 48 to 72 hours before you work the same muscles again.

Advanced Weight Training

After a few months of working out, you will be ready to do more work with weights to continue your progress. Ways to do that include performing more sets of each exercise as well as more exercises. Depending on your schedule, you may also want to increase your number of training days, possibly using a split routine. This involves working your upper body twice a week and your lower body twice a week for a total of four training days a week.

You will be surprised at the speed of your progress because of the new, healthy way you are eating – mainly all the quality calories you are taking in. Steve H., an avid weight trainer, was amazed at how much his strength levels increased after following the program. "I came to Lean Bodies to lose bodyfat, and I did. But I stayed at the same weight because I gained lean body mass, which boosted my strength. I'm now doing twice as many repetitions on bench presses."

Sticking To Your Plan

Many people join a gym, buy an exercise bike, or sign up for aerobic dancing, and then work out with all the zeal of an Olympic athlete in hard training – only to drop out weeks later. The exercise routine turns into a memory, kept alive by running shoes, tennis gear, exercise videos, or barbells, all gathering dust.

Sadly, only one American in five gets regular exercise.[20] Of those who do exercise regularly, most are adults. In fact, youth fitness is on the decline. While Mom and Dad are out jogging, their kids are probably at home watching TV and munching on junk food – a behavior that could establish lifelong patterns of inactivity.

Health professionals report that of all those who start an exercise program, about half will drop out within six months to a year.[21] In addition, an overwhelming number of would-be exercisers may not make it past the first two weeks. So what is the problem? Why aren't more people jogging miles, pumping iron, swimming laps? Simply put: motivation.

On the surface, exercise is not a particularly motivating activity. It hurts. It takes time. It can be boring, frustrating, even embarrassing – especially if you think your body is less-than-perfect and you do not like to be seen in leotards or gym shorts. Plus, when the desired results fail to materialize fast enough, you give up in despair. Exercise, you conclude, is only for fanatics. So why even try?

You try because you want to look better, feel better, live better. You have already read that exercise enhances your life – physically and mentally. Deep down, you want the motivation that will lead to better health. Your problem is how to get motivated and stay that way.

Secrets of Exercise Success

More than anything else, success at sticking to an exercise program depends on your nutritional status. Remember: Food is fuel. Too many people make the mistake of working out – and working out hard – without enough gas in the tank. They run out of energy, and as a result, they run out of motivation to continue.

This is what happened to Lee W., a former fat child and an anorexic teen. A year before starting our program, Lee lost 25 pounds, and she did it by exercising on a stairclimbing machine. After working out, she would drink a diet soda and eat a handful of candy. Lunch was always a salad; dinner, French fries. This diet added up to less than 1000 calories a day.

Lee's energy levels would dip so low because of lack of fuel that she would crash with fatigue. After a year of this, she started attending my classes. At the time, Lee was what I call a "thin/fat:" she weighed 110 pounds but had a bodyfat percentage of 26 percent.

By the end of six weeks, she had lost 3-percent bodyfat. She continued to lose, eventually reaching a bodyfat percentage of 18.

Her energy levels were so high and sustained that she decided to compete in a vertical climb marathon, in which competitors run up the stairs of a skyscraper. Now she's a dedicated vertical climber and marathoner — all because of proper nutrition.

Joe O. had a similar experience. He came to his first Lean Bodies class weighing 385 pounds with more than 40-percent bodyfat. "Five days after starting the program, I began to feel so good that I decided to start exercising again," he says.

He kept exercising, month after month after month, always using the stationary bike. "Never in my life had I stuck to a workout program so consistently."

Joe entered a national competition sponsored by a chain of health clubs to which he belonged. To his amazement, he won the stationary bike competition, turning in the best time of all the other entrants across the United States.

"Before, I could have never done this. In fact, if someone had told me I would win a national competition, I wouldn't have believed it."

Joe eats about 3,500 calories a day, has lost more than 50 pounds, and is down to 20-percent bodyfat.

Exercise success also depends on your mental attitude. If you look at all your failed attempts to get in shape as just that — failures — then you are bound to repeat your stop/start patterns of exercise. Instead, congratulate yourself for all the times you have tried. Along the way, you probably discovered many types of exercise that really did not work for you, either because you did not enjoy them or you physically could not perform them. Just the same, begin to think of those attempts as experiments that are moving you closer to your objective: a time when exercise is no longer a struggle, when exercise is a permanent part of your lifestyle. Reaching that objective requires some changes on your part – changes in the way you think, changes in the way you live. But the process of changing from an inactive lifestyle to an active one can only be positive. It is change that will let you live more fully.

It may reassure you to know that change takes place in an erratic way. Your track record will show a few false starts, along with some sustained runs. If you are not prepared for the false starts, you will panic and want to give up. As long as you are aware that you will have setbacks, you will be easier on yourself. Remember: Progress is built on perseverance.

Enjoyment has plenty to do with your level of dedication too. The more satisfaction you get from exercise, the greater your motivation to continue. When you are a dedicated exerciser, exercise is a pleasure rather than a duty.

Many successful exercisers have a supportive network of instructors, coaches, friends, or spouses who keep them going even when they feel like giving up. Even research suggests the importance of support in sustaining motivation. Studies show that beginners are more successful when they work out with others, and people who exercise in groups have twice the adherence of those who try it alone. Exercise partnerships are proving to be an important element in cementing dedication.

When you are dedicated to exercise, you work hard at it, without excuses, without apologies. You feel compelled to master the activity and explore your own physical potential, whatever the activity may be.

CHAPTER NINE

¶ *Key Points*

• Aerobic exercise is the only type of physical activity that directly burns bodyfat.

• An indirect way to burn fat is by weight training, which develops muscle tissue, the body's most metabolically active tissue. The more muscle you have, the better your body can burn fat.

• Exercise is proving to be an important preventive factor in many diseases, some of them life-threatening.

• There are many types of exercise programs from which to choose, each offering various fitness benefits.

• Exercise motivation can stay high with the proper nutrition and a program that is convenient, enjoyable, and tailored to individual objectives.

10

❦ *Nutritional Needs of Exercisers and Athletes*

ROLAND J., a gym owner and former national competitive bodybuilder, was losing weight, but not bodyfat, when he came to Lean Bodies for help. "After quitting competitive bodybuilding, I tried to train with some intensity to keep myself in good condition," he explains. "But with all my training, I couldn't understand why I was losing muscle mass."

Roland was training above what his nutritional level would allow. In other words, he was not adequately feeding his body to properly drive the catabolism/anabolism cycle. If you remember, exercise breaks muscle down. To repair and build it, you need protein and other nutrients. Roland was simply not getting enough of these nutrients to support this process. Additionally, he was hypoglycemic and would experience dizziness, cold sweats, and mood alterations when his blood sugar dipped.

Once Roland increased his calories, including protein, and began eating more frequently, things started to change. In eight weeks, he gained 20 pounds of muscle and his hypoglycemia was under complete control. Today, Roland eats an average of 3,500 calories daily, spread out over six meals a day. He works out with weights five times a week and does aerobics four times a week.

Not everyone who comes to Lean Bodies wants to lose bodyfat. Many, like Roland, want to gain lean mass (muscle) so they can look better, feel more energized, and improve their sports performance.

When people want to put on mass, one of the first questions I ask is "How much protein are you eating?" Not surprisingly, their protein intake is usually too low to build lean mass or even maintain good health.

Take Holly B., age 41, for example. She had her eye on becoming a triathlete yet subsisted on two meals a day of fruit and yogurt. ("I thought I was eating a healthful diet," she says.) The problem was, Holly had no energy. How could she possibly compete in a triathlon?

I told her that triathlons were out of the question until she started eating more protein, along with more meals and some nutritional supplements. Six months later, after committing to the program, she competed in her first triathlon. Now she's a confirmed triathlete – and a confirmed "lean body."

More and more, research in clinical nutrition is showing that active people, including athletes, have increased requirements for protein – far above the current RDA of 0.8 grams/kg body weight per day for the average person. A study by Peter W.R. Lemon, Ph.D., one of the leading researchers in the area of protein requirements for athletes, found that endurance athletes need 25 to 50 percent more protein than the RDA.[1]

Unfortunately, the RDA was developed from studies of sedentary individuals and does not take into account the needs of more active people. In one study, weight lifters who were eating 250 percent of the RDA for protein still showed a negative nitrogen balance (this is a measurement of whether you are gaining or losing lean mass). In another study, after protein was increased from 255 percent to 438 percent of the RDA, weight lifters gained muscle mass.[2]

For building lean mass, the best source of protein is lean animal protein. It is more "insulinogenic" than vegetable proteins; in other words, it produces more insulin, and insulin is an important anabolic (growth-producing) hormone. Animal proteins also elevate levels of somatomedin, an insulin-like growth factor. This response is not produced by vegetable proteins.[3]

Is Too Much Protein Harmful?

Among some nutrition experts, there is a widespread opinion that excess dietary protein and phosphorus (a mineral found in animal proteins) lead to urinary calcium loss. Yet long-term studies do not support this. In fact, numerous studies have been done showing that high dietary protein does not cause calcium loss. In one study, for example, nine men ate a high meat diet for several months, and urinary calcium did not increase – except in one subject who was taking a medication known to cause calcium loss.[4]

Dietary proteins such as meat and milk are high in phosphorus, and this, along with protein, has been blamed for calcium loss. In another study, a daily 2,000 mg dose of phosphorus had no adverse effects on the use of calcium by the body. In fact, phosphorus has been used with other therapeutic measures to increase bone mass in patients with osteoporosis.[5]

Gaining Lean Mass

If you are like most exercisers and athletes, one of your goals is to gain muscle. The more muscle you have the stronger you are, the better you perform, and the less prone you are to athletic injuries. As I have already emphasized, muscle helps you burn bodyfat more efficiently – as well as keep that fat off. The Lean Bodies program, with its multiple meals approach to eating, works beautifully for people who want to gain muscle.

Barry E., 44, is a good example. He is what you would call a classic "ectomorph," tall, lean, not too muscular. "I was already in reasonably good shape when I started the program. I didn't really want to reduce. My body composition, however, had begun to change as I got older. I had a little more bodyfat and a little less lean mass. I wanted to reverse that process by gaining lean mass and strength.

"Athletic performance is important to me, too. As a tennis player, I play guys 15 to 20 years younger than I am. Because I want to keep up with them, I decided to take better care of myself with nutrition."

Barry is well on his way to achieving his goals. Already he has reduced his bodyfat by 2 percent and gained several pounds of muscle.

If gaining muscle mass is your main goal, here is an example of a Lean Bodies meal plan that can help you:

Gainers Menu*

Breakfast
4 large scrambled egg whites
2 scoops (2 oz.) carbohydrate supplement, mixed with water
1½ cups oatmeal
1 cup skim milk
2 tbsp. MCT oil

Mock Meal
2 scoops (2 oz.) carbohydrate supplement and 1 scoop (1 oz.) protein powder mixed with water, Crystal Light, or sugar-free Tang

Lunch
6 oz. chicken breast
12 oz. sweet potato

The nutrient values of menus are based on use of Pro-Carb™ (protein/carbohydrate supplement) and Hi-Protein Powder™ (Protein Powder), manufactured by parrillo Performance. use of other supplements may yield different nutrient values.

1 cup black-eyed peas
1 cup green beans
2 tbsp. MCT oil

Mini-Meal
2 scoops (2 oz.) carbohydrate supplement and 1 scoop (1 oz.) protein
powder mixed with water, Crystal Light, or sugar-free Tang
2 oz. tuna
Brown rice (cook ⅔ cup to yield proper portion)
2 tbsp. MCT oil

Dinner
6 oz. halibut
14 oz. potato
2 cups broccoli
2 cups corn

TOTAL DAILY NUTRIENTS: 4,151 calories; 226.1 g protein; 594.8 g carbohydrate; 23.1 g fat; 1,105 mg sodium; 8,063 mg potassium; and 1,299 mg calcium.
Note: If you require a specific daily amount of calcium, ask your physician if it may
be obtained by increased dairy, deep green leafy vegetables and/or a calcium/
magnesium supplement.

Other Performance Nutrients

So far, I have covered the protein needs of exercisers and athletes
– mainly because this is a misunderstood and largely uncharted area
of sports nutrition. Active people need more protein – but they need
more of other nutrients as well. This is easily accomplished by increasing calories (the right kind of calories).

You may not be aware of it, but the high-calorie method of eating
is really nothing new to elite athletes. Long-distance runners, for

example, may consume up to 5,000 calories a day. During their training season, swimmers may have to eat up to 6,000 calories just to maintain their body weight. And, competitive bodybuilders often eat up to 10,000 calories during the off-season to support heavier training and corresponding increases in muscle mass.

It is surprising that many active people put their exercise and training programs ahead of proper nutrition, when it should be the other way around. Harold D., a Ph.D. and a psychotherapist, age 43, had always been athletic, but as he puts it, "I had not ever seriously focused on the nutritional aspects of fitness." As Harold discovered, good nutrition enhanced his already active lifestyle. After attending my Lean Bodies classes, he told me, "In the last three months, I have lost about 30 pounds, four inches around my waist, and I cannot remember feeling this good in the past 15 years."

For active people like Harold and serious athletes, inadequate nutrition can hurt health and impair performance. Olympic hopeful Juanita E. runs track. As she explains it: "What you weigh on the day of your race is very important to how well you perform. I felt like I knew what my best race weight was, and I would typically cut calories to drop down to that weight.

"Cutting calories, however, led to a series of health problems, including mononucleosis and orthopedic injuries. Eventually, I recovered from those, only to start having dizzy spells – to the point of passing out. My physician did blood tests and discovered that not only was I hypoglycemic, but also that I had the Epstein Barre virus."

Juanita traveled to Salt Lake City to train at the U.S. Olympic Committee training facility. It was there that she first heard that athletes should be eating in the 4,000-calories-a-day range. "But most of the time, I'd still eat only 1,200 calories a day," she says. "By the end of my stay though, I had built up to 3,000, but a lot of those calories were processed carbohydrates. After returning home, I was still dogged by injury, namely plantar fascitis [an overuse injury that causes pain in the heel or arch of the foot]. My body was breaking down, and I felt it was all food related. That's when I decided to go to Lean Bodies."

Today, Juanita eats an average of 3,000 calories a day, sometimes more, and her weight has stabilized within a pound or two of where she wants it to be. She reports that she has more energy than ever to train.

The high calorie diets of athletes are typically loaded with carbohydrates – and justifiably so. Carbohydrates are converted into glycogen, the stored fuel in your muscles. As you begin exercising, the release of adrenalin signals the breakdown of muscle glycogen into glucose. Your muscles start using glucose as fuel to contract. If your muscles are well-stocked with glycogen, you have enough fuel to run on.

If you are an exerciser or athlete who does not take in enough calories every day, particularly starchy carbohydrates, then you are headed for trouble. Hard training and competition use up glycogen, and when that happens, endurance and performance drop. But by eating the right foods throughout the day, you are constantly fueling yourself to prevent fatigue from setting in. It is important to add that, following a training session, muscles are most receptive to synthesizing new glycogen – as long as you take in carbohydrates after your workout. An easy and excellent way to do this is by drinking the maltodextrin-based carbohydrate beverage used in the Lean Bodies mock meal.

As far as other carbohydrates are concerned, a daily Lean Bodies menu contains 65 percent carbohydrates – exactly the right amount to prevent glycogen depletion.

Vitamins and Minerals

As an exerciser or athlete, you may need extra help in the form of vitamin and mineral supplementation to support the demands of training. Certain vitamins and minerals are depleted with exercise and training, and these include:

B-complex vitamins. The members of the B-complex family to be concerned about are riboflavin, thiamine, and B_6. If you are an active woman, you may require more riboflavin, and your need for thiamine goes up in proportion to how much energy you use. Other research has shown that the body draws heavily upon stores of vitamin B_6 during aerobic exercise such as running and cycling. Remember that if you use vitamin supplements, the B-complex family must be taken together, rather than in single doses of B-vitamins.

Iron. This vital mineral can be lost through perspiration, and in female athletes, through blood flow during menstruation. Any exerciser or athlete following a vegetarian diet is at risk for an iron deficiency, because iron from plant sources (nonheme iron) is not well absorbed. Certain athletes – namely dancers, wrestlers, and gymnasts – often severely restrict calories to keep their weight low, and this practice can lead to an iron deficiency, as well as to other nutritional problems.

The iron status of endurance athletes has often been called into question. Many researchers have found iron depletion and iron deficiencies in these athletes. Several years ago, an interesting study examined the iron status of 50 endurance athletes (31 men and 19 women) competing in the 1988 Ironman Triathlon in Hawaii. Remarkably, only two of the triathletes (both women) in the study had a true iron deficiency. The healthy iron status among the others may have been a result of diet, according to the researchers. As they noted, "Triathletes are generally conscious of good nutrition, a trend that is reflected in this study by the adequacy of iron intake through both food and supplementation."[6]

Chromium. This important trace mineral appears to play a role in fighting bodyfat and building lean mass. In one study, a group of men took chromium picolinate (a supplemental form of the mineral), while a control group took a placebo. Those who took chromium were able to significantly increase lean mass in 42 days. By the end of the study, the chromium-supplemented group had gained an average of 5.9 pounds. In addition, they dropped their average total bodyfat from 15.8 percent to 12.2 percent – a 22-percent loss in bodyfat. Lean mass and bodyfat percentage changes in the placebo group were not significant.[7]

Electrolytes. These are sodium, potassium, magnesium, and chloride – the minerals that keep your fluid balance in check by regulating the water inside and outside your cells. Deficiencies of potassium and magnesium are often found in athletes. Drains on potassium typically occur as a result of profuse sweating during hot weather training, and deficiencies bring on fatigue. Similarly, a low-magnesium diet can lower your endurance during training. This is because magnesium is involved in controlling muscle contraction and converting carbohydrates to energy.

Zinc. Studies of marathon runners have shown that training tends to deplete zinc stores, indicating that these athletes may have to keep an eye on their intake of this important mineral. Fortunately though, a high-calorie diet supplies all the zinc a hard-training athlete needs. Vegetarian athletes need to be cautious, though, because they are missing out on an important source of zinc: lean animal proteins.

Metabolic Optimizers

These are a relatively new class of natural supplements believed to enhance athletic performance, though the jury is still out on whether some claims are true. As supplements, metabolic optimizers are typically used by athletes who wish to increase lean muscle mass, improve strength, and enhance endurance. Here are several of the popular metabolic optimizers:

Aspartates. The increased rate of ammonia production by the body has been suggested by researchers to be one of the causes of the fatigue that accompanies intense exercise. Aspartates are involved in turning excess ammonia to urea, which is then eliminated from the body. Studies have shown that potassium and magnesium aspartates increase the endurance of swimming rats, possibly by producing lower-than-normal rises in ammonia concentration.

A recent study looked at this effect in seven healthy men, all competitors in various sports, who were tested on a bicycle ergometer. At intervals during a 24-hour period prior to the test, four of the men took a total of five grams of potassium and five grams of magnesium aspartate. The others took a placebo. During the test, they pedaled at 50 rpm at a moderately high intensity. Blood samples were taken prior to, during, and after the test. A week later, the men participated in the same experiment but the conditions were reversed.

Blood ammonia concentrations for the aspartate-supplemented group were found to be significantly lower than that of the placebo group. And, endurance was boosted by about 14 percent in the aspartate group. On average, the aspartate group cycled a total of 88 minutes before reaching a point of exhaustion, whereas the other group cycled about 75 minutes until exhaustion. The researchers noted that "the results of this study would suggest that potassium and magnesium aspartate are useful in increasing endurance performance."[8]

Aspartate supplements are usually available in health food stores and sports fitness centers.

Branched-chain amino acids. A popular bodybuilding supplement, these amino acids (leucine, isoleucine, and valine) act as nitrogen carriers that assist the muscles in synthesizing other amino acids to aid in muscular growth. They stimulate the production of insulin, which allows circulating blood sugar to be absorbed by the muscle cells and used as a source of energy.

Supplemental branched-chain amino acids have been getting some attention in research circles. In a study at Old Dominion University in Norfolk, Virginia, researchers observed the effect of amino acid supplementation on the endurance of highly trained athletes. These athletes were divided into two groups: One group took about 14 grams of branched-chain amino acids (isoleucine, leucine, and valine, which are burned for energy in the muscles when glycogen stores are low), and the control group took a placebo. Both groups ate the same diet, which consisted of protein and carbohydrates, while following their usual training routine.

When tested at the end of a two-week period, the athletes who took the supplements had actually gained lean mass. Not only that, they ran approximately one minute per mile faster than the control group. Blood tests suggested that the supplements may preserve muscle glycogen by mobilizing more fat for energy.[9]

Desiccated Liver. For decades, desiccated liver has been a popular nutritional supplement. Available in tablet or powdered form, this product is made from whole Argentina beef liver that has been vacuum dried at low temperatures to preserve the nutrient content. Desiccated liver is rich in vitamins A, B, C, and D; heme iron; calcium; and phosphorus. It has four times the nutritional value as the same amount of cooked whole liver.

In animal studies, desiccated liver has been shown to enhance endurance and increase strength. In a study by Dr. B.H. Ershoff, three groups of rats were fed controlled diets for three months. One group consumed a basic diet supplemented with vitamins and minerals; the second group ate the same diet, along with B-complex vitamins and brewer's yeast; and the third group ate the basic diet, supplemented with desiccated liver. The rats were placed in water to see how long they could swim before drowning. Group one swam an average of 13.2 minutes; and group two, an average of 13.4 minutes. Remarkably, the desiccated liver-supplemented rats were still swimming at the end of two hours – 10 times longer than the other two groups.[10]

MCT Oil. Because of its structure, MCT oil is absorbed more quickly and efficiently than ordinary dietary fats and is used by the body as energy fuel. Since it is rapidly oxidized by the body, MCT oil is rarely stored as bodyfat. Athletes use MCT oil as a source of extra calories (114 per tablespoon) so that they can train longer and harder – and put on more muscle mass as a result. People on the Lean Bodies program who take MCT oil love it because of the energy it gives them. They have even nicknamed it "liquid energy."

Supplemental Amino Acid Growth Hormone Releasers. Studies have shown that the amino acids arginine, pyroglutamate, and lysine elevate the level of human growth hormone (HGH) in the blood. One study demonstrated that a combination of arginine (1,200 mg) and lysine (1,200 mg) triggered the release of growth hormone in humans up to 794 percent.[11]

As previously mentioned, do not take nutritional supplements, including metabolic optimizers, without first consulting your physician.

Meeting the Nutritional Demands of Training

In the Lean Bodies program, I encourage participants to take up more active lifestyles. As several of the case studies in this book show, many people have taken my advice, going on to become marathoners, triathletes, and dedicated exercisers.

As you become more active, you must continually scrutinize your nutrition. With a sustained increase in activity, there should be a corresponding increase in your calories. Remember: Protein builds and repairs muscles, and carbohydrates give your body energy during workouts. Eat more of these foods as you increase your training. And where supplementation is concerned, vitamins and minerals, as well as metabolic optimizers, provide excellent insurance against deficiencies caused by training and may even enhance your athletic performance.

☘ *Key Points*

• The protein needs of active people are higher than the current Recommended Daily Allowance (RDA).

• Protein is the primary nutrient involved in building lean mass.

• Exercisers and athletes need plenty of carbohydrates, which can be rapidly depleted by long, intense training sessions.

• Exercisers and athletes may need additional nutrients in the form of vitamin and mineral supplements, such as B-complex vitamins, iron, chromium, electrolytes, and trace minerals such as zinc.

• Some nutrients, known as metabolic optimizers, may enhance athletic performance. These include aspartates, branched-chain amino acids, desiccated liver, MCT oil, and supplemental growth hormone releasers.

11

¶ *Leaner and Fitter for a Lifetime*

AS A FORMER DIETER, you may have already experienced what 95 percent of other dieters have experienced: The weight is regained, with interest, once you stop dieting. And the main reason is the slowdown in metabolism as a result of cut-calorie dieting. With the Lean Bodies program, there is no slowdown. Instead, there is a speeding up of the metabolism. This means you can handle a variety of foods better than ever before – and without fear of regaining bodyfat. Once you start reintroducing other foods back into your meals, you use the calories up, rather than store them as fat.

Another problem with "diets" is that they're temporary. You can't stay on them forever. You'd either get ill from lack of nutrients, bored with the limited food choices, or both. The Lean Bodies program is one that you can stay on. A low bodyfat percentage, lots of calories, a ton of energy, better health – who would want to give those up? I asked some of our lean bodies if they felt the program could become part of their lifestyle forever. Here's what they said:

"I just got on it and stayed on it. I'm never hungry. I'm eating all I can eat. Right now, I'm at 5,000 calories a day."

"It is a lifestyle. My only regret is that I didn't know about it earlier."

"I have more of a sense of well-being. I've learned how to eat to fuel my body. I can stay on this program the rest of my life."

"I have made a lifestyle change, and it was easy."

"I'm at a point now where I can 'cheat' – and not regain bodyfat."

"I will never return to a low-calorie diet."

"I go to bed full, and I wake up hungry. I can't imagine ever dieting again."

"The program is easy to stick to, because you're not starving yourself."

"At first, I honestly thought I was going to be a dropout. But now the program has become a part of me."

"This is the first 'diet' I've ever stayed on."

"When people ask me, 'How's your diet going?' I tell them 'It's not a diet. It's a life change.' I'll be eating this way the rest of my life."

After the first seven weeks of following the Lean Bodies program, you'll be ready to start adding foods such as pasta and breads (the whole grain varieties are best) and lean red meats back into your menus. Keep in mind that your metabolism is faster than ever before – after all, you're eating 2,000, 3,000, or more calories a day so you can handle these additions. Here's a sample menu to show you how to plan meals with additional foods*:

Breakfast
3 large scrambled egg whites
1 cup oatmeal
4 oz. nonfat yogurt
½ tbsp. MCT oil

Mock Meal
2 scoops (2 oz.) carbohydrate supplement mixed with water,
    Crystal Light, or sugar-free Tang

The nutrient values of menus are based on use of Pro-Carb™ (protein/carbohydrate supplement) and Hi-Protein Powder™ (protein powder), manufactured by Parrillo Performance. Use of other supplements may yield different nutrient values.

Lunch

6 oz. chicken breast on a whole grain bun

1 cup black-eyed peas

1 cup green beans

4 oz. frozen yogurt

Mini-Meal

1 scoop (2 oz.) carbohydrate supplement mixed with water,
    Crystal Light, or sugar-free Tang

1 medium green apple

Dinner

4 oz. cod

Whole grain pasta (cook 4 oz. dry weight to yield proper portion)

1 cup green beans

TOTAL DAILY NUTRIENTS: 2,126 calories; 147.4 g protein; 334.9 g carbo-hydrate; 17.6 g fat; 1,465 mg sodium; and 3,924 mg potassium, 990 mg calcium. Note: If you require a specific daily amount of calcium, ask your physician if it may be obtained by increased dairy, deep green leafy vegetables and/or a calcium/ magnesium supplement.

Planned Cheats

Before Lean Bodies, there might have been a time in your dieting life when every goody seemed to turn right into bodyfat, no matter how small the portion. And you probably ate a lot of goodies, especially after falling off the "diet wagon." On this program, there's no wagon to fall off of. In the first place, you're eating more calories and more food than you probably ever have in your life. You're not hungry so you don't feel like "pigging out." **Once you've achieved your bodyfat percentage goal, if you do feel like having some ice cream, pie, cookies, cake, or pizza, go ahead and eat it.** Metabolically, now you can handle it. As you start experiencing how well your body uses food, you won't feel guilty about eating foods that are forbidden on most diets. **Remember too that exercise is a key component of weight control because it expends calories for energy — so maintain your level of activity.**

I recommend to people that they practice something I call a "planned cheat." Simply put, this means planning to eat a treat on a certain day, at a certain time – without eating on impulse. Impulsive eating leads to more impulsive eating, not to mention a pile of guilt. When you plan your "cheats," you give yourself permission to eat, and there's no guilt.

"I did not cheat the first seven weeks," says James J., who came to Lean Bodies weighing 260 pounds (he's six-foot-one) and lost 55 pounds in four months. "But now I do cheat occasionally. Because my metabolism is so fast, I can handle the food. Best of all, I'm still losing weight." Incidentally, James is losing bodyfat on 4,300 calories a day.

I do not want to give you the impression that you can go on planned cheats every day, however. That would defeat the whole purpose of Lean Bodies. While keeping your calories up, you must continue to eat lean proteins, starchy carbohydrates, lean, fibrous vegetables, and essential fatty acids – in the ratio of protein, 25 percent; carbohydrates, 65 percent; and fats, 10 percent.

Optimum Fueling

As you achieve your desired bodyfat percentage and weight, you will reach a caloric ceiling at which you can maintain those desirable levels. Here is a formula you can use that will help you calculate the number of calories you need each day for optimum fueling and maintenance:

BW = *Ideal Projected Body Weight*

BMR = *Basal Metabolic Rate*

VMA = *Voluntary Muscular Activity*

SDA = *Specific Dynamic Action*

BW / 2.2 = BW (*kg) x .9 (for women) = Women's BW kg

BW kg x 24 hrs = BMR

BMR x .75 (** This number can vary depending on your activity level) = VMA

BMR + VMA = Calories x .1 = SDA

BMR + VMA + SDA = Calories for Optimal Fueling

Losing Fat / Gaining Health

We have an expression in our Lean Bodies classes that goes like this: "losing fat, gaining health." As I've said throughout this book, many of the people I work with have been able to regain their health by following the program. And that's the amazing thing about good nutrition: its impact on health. Did you know, for instance, that five of the 10 most life-threatening diseases in our country could be improved by changes in the diet? That's right. Susceptibility to heart disease, stroke, diabetes, certain forms of cancer, and gastrointestinal illnesses can be lessened by better nutrition.[1]

But, one of the most extraordinary cases I've ever encountered as a clinical nutritionist was Patty E., age 44, who was diagnosed by her doctor as having Meniere's Syndrome. This is a disease that affects the inner ear and is characterized by recurrent attacks of dizziness, nausea, vomiting, and gradual loss of hearing. The only treatment for Meniere's Syndrome is a low-salt diet and diuretics. She came to the Lean Bodies program to get help in monitoring her sodium intake.

---

*A kilogram (kg) equals 2.21 pounds

**If you are a sedentary, use .50 here; moderately active (you exercise 3 to 4 times a week, doing aerobics), .65; and very active, 1.

"A month later, I went to my doctor [a Meniere's Syndrome specialist] to have a hearing test. He was shocked. I was the first Meniere's patient he had seen in 27 years whose hearing had actually improved! He was so amazed that he wants me to come in to talk to other Meniere's patients about how I'm eating."

Patty is off medication completely – and she's exercising, something her doctors told her she would never be able to do. Incidentally, Patty has lost 16 pounds. "I look the same as I did when I was in my twenties," she says.

It's difficult to pinpoint exactly how and why Patty's condition improved so dramatically. But even so, sometimes nutrition, for whatever reason, turns out to be the best medicine.

In reality, nutrition works hand in hand with medicine to produce the best possible outcome. A good example is Kathy C., who, upon turning 40, began to have hot flashes, accompanied by high blood pressure, severe anxiety, and panic attacks. Her internist diagnosed her condition as an endocrine system disorder. The endocrine system is made up of ductless glands (such as the adrenal and pituitary glands) that secrete hormones internally.

The results of her blood test showed that her blood sugar was dropping drastically throughout the day, most likely because of hormonal imbalances. "So Cliff had me eat every two hours, with more emphasis on protein and vitamin supplements," Kathy says.

"In three days, I began to feel better by cutting out the sugar, which was having an adverse effect on my hormonal system. And even though I don't have a weight problem, I eventually lost three pounds. Once my blood sugar was under control, I began medical treatment for my hormonal imbalances and blood pressure elevation. Now I feel great."

I mention Kathy's case because it's a great example of how nutrition and medicine, working together, make a great team.

Healthy Aging

Are you 40 going on 75 or 75 going on 40? While you are thinking about your answer, let me tell you about one of the most remarkable people I've ever met. About 40 years ago, David S., a businessman, was putting in long hours in his family's jewelry business trying to turn a profit at one particular store. When his weight ballooned to 203 pounds (David is five-foot-nine), he decided to do something about it. He modified his diet to include more nutritious food, and he started exercising. At first, he worked out three times week, but then progressed to seven times a week. To this day, he has kept that regimen up.

Today, David is over 80 years old, and he's one of the fittest, most energetic people I know. His exercise schedule is beyond belief. In the morning, he starts out with stretches, 200 sit-ups, dips and chins, two sets of biceps curls, a set of leg presses with 210 pounds, abdominal twists – and then he does a circuit of 10 Nautilus machines. After that, he works out on the treadmill. But he's not finished yet. David then plays three games of racquetball. By the way, he's the Golden Age Racquetball Champion in the United States. Also, his resting heart rate is 56 (that's healthy!), and at his age, he's put on six pounds of pure muscle.

David's nutrition is as impressive as his exercise. David eats whole grains, lots of vegetables and complex carbohydrates, fish, chicken, and lean red meat once a week. His doctor says he has the body of a 30-year-old, and believe me, he looks like one.

You might think that David has some secret for staying young or that he's gifted genetically. But for half his life now, David has lived a consistently healthy lifestyle, eating highly nutritious foods and working out vigorously seven days a week. I believe that there has to be some connection. Does this mean that you can stay in great physical and mental shape longer if you follow David's example? According to recent studies, it looks like the answer is "yes." For example:

• Diets rich in potassium appear to have a protective effect against hypertension, the major cause of strokes, according to research. Potassium has also been shown to reduce the blood pressures of hypertensive patients. The reasons for this are unclear, yet may be associated with potassium's involvement in physiological systems that regulate blood pressure.[2]

Essential fatty acids (EFAs) also seem to reduce blood pressure. In a study of healthy people in Italy, Finland, and the United States, researchers found more hypertensives among Finns than among the other populations. The dietary difference was that the Finns ate more saturated fats and less polyunsaturated fats than the others, whose diets were high in linoleic acid (a polyunsaturate). When a group of Finns (ages 40 to 50) consumed a low-fat diet high in polyunsaturated fats and low in saturated fats, their blood pressures dropped significantly.[3]

• Antioxidants continue to prove themselves as anti-aging nutrients. In one study, 45 elderly subjects took an antioxidant formulation of betacarotene, vitamins C and E, selenium, and zinc for one year. At regular periods, the researchers checked something called "lipid peroxides" in all of the subjects. These are products from the oxidation of fats and are good indicators of the level of oxidation taking place in the body. Oxidation is the corrosion of cellular membranes that is thought to be responsible for aging.

Before the study began, the elderly subjects had high levels of lipid peroxidation. After being on the antioxidant formula for three months, the subjects were compared with a control group of healthy young adults. The results showed that the elderly's level of lipid peroxidation fell to levels lower than that of the control group and remained there for the rest of the study.[4]

• The ability of the cells in your body to synthesize new protein is critical for bolstering immunity and warding off infection. You can become protein-deficient very quickly. Case in point: The effect of a nine-day low-protein diet was studied in six young and six elderly (average age 72) healthy subjects. At the end of the study period, nitrogen balance and levels of certain blood compounds were measured. In both groups, nitrogen balance decreased (nitrogen balance indicates whether you're losing or gaining lean mass). Most significant was the reduced level of transferrin in the blood. Transferrin ferries iron to sites of need in the body. Studies have shown that when transferrin levels fall, possibly due to a protein deficiency, the immune system is weakened. The authors emphasized that a low-calorie, low-protein diet can increase vulnerability to both infection and chronic disease, especially in the elderly.[5]

• An active lifestyle enhances functional capacity in later years. That's the finding of a study of older men and women who underwent exercise testing during the 1985 World Masters Games in Toronto, Canada. When the subjects were tested on cycle ergometers, their aerobic power was above average, when compared to nonathletes of the same age, and matched that of sedentary 25-year-olds.[6]

• Exercise, including weight training and aerobics, can improve quality of life among the elderly. In a six-month study of 56 men and women (age 70 to 79), researchers compared the effects of weight training or a walk/jog program to the effects of no exercise. The exercisers improved their strength and cardiovascular fitness dramatically. Studies of older people who weight train are showing that this form of exercise builds strength, thus helping them stay active longer and live more independent lives.[7]

• Longevity may be positively influenced by exercise, according to a major study of 16,936 Harvard alumni. In the study, researchers found that those alumni who lived an active lifestyle, with regular exercise, lived up to two years longer than those who were sedentary.[8]

Your Personal Quality Of Life

It's difficult to predict how you will age. After all, you are different from anyone else, with your own biochemical individuality. But it's clear that many elements of nutrition and fitness are within your control – elements that can enhance your quality of life. Naturally, the earlier you start on a healthy lifestyle, the better your health may be in later years. But it's never too late to start.

By now, I hope you are convinced of the power of nutrition in your health. If nothing else, I hope you believe that "diets" are a no-win proposition when it comes to losing fat and gaining health. Changing your biochemistry so that you stay lean and fit is an ongoing process. Like an athlete striving for the next goal, you must constantly strive to make yourself more efficient – with a well-tuned metabolism, a healthy body, and a positive perspective. By giving your body all the resources it needs, you will reach those goals.

❧ *Key Points*

• Because the Lean Bodies program speeds up your metabolism, you can now handle a variety of foods – without regaining bodyfat.

• After seven weeks on the Lean Bodies program, you may start adding foods such as breads and pasta back into your diet.

• "Planned cheats" give you permission to eat other foods.

• Nutrition has the power to reduce the risks of heart disease, stroke, diabetes, certain forms of cancer, and gastrointestinal diseases.

• As you get older, you can stay in excellent physical and mental shape with proper nutrition and an active lifestyle.

Notes

References

References

Chapter 1: It's Time to Eat!

1. Geissler, C.A., Miller, D.S., and Shah, M. "The Daily Metabolic Rate of the Post-Obese and the Lean." *The American Journal of Clinical Nutrition* (1987); 45: 914-22.

2. Blackburn, G.L., Wilson, G.T., Kanders, B.S., et al. "Weight Cycling: The Experience of Human Dieters." *The American Journal of Clinical Nutrition* (1989); 49: 1105-1109.

3. Schelkin, P.H. "The Risks of Riding the Weight Loss Rollercoaster." *The Physician and Sportsmedicine* (June 1991); vol. 19, no. 6: 153.

4. Lissner, L., Odell, P.M., D'Agostino, R.B., et al. "Variability of Body Weight and Health Outcomes in the Framingham Population." *The New England Journal of Medicine* (June 27, 1991); vol. 324, no. 26: 1839-1844.

5. Liddle, R.A., Goldstein, R.B., Saxton, J. "Gallstone Formation during Weight-Reduction Dieting." *Archives of Internal Medicine* (1989); vol. 149: 1750-1753.

6. Schelkin, P.H. "The Risks of Riding the Weight Loss Rollercoaster." *The Physician and Sportsmedicine* (June 1991); vol. 19, no. 6: 150-151.

7. Felig, P. "Very-Low-Calorie Protein Diets." *The New England Journal of Medicine* (March 1, 1984); vol. 310, no. 9: 589-591.

8. Greenwood-Robinson, M. "Danger Zone Dieting." *MuscleMag International* (December 1988/January 1989): 64-67.

9. Yates, A., Leehey K., and Shisslak, C.M. "Running – An Analogue of Anorexia?" *The New England Journal of Medicine* (February 3, 1983); vol. 308: 251-255.

10. Jenkins, D.J.A., Wolever, T.M.S., Vuksan, V., et al. "Nibbling Versus Gorging: Metabolic Advantages of Increased Meal Frequency." *The New England Journal of Medicine* (October 5, 1989); vol. 321, no. 14: 929-931.

11. University of Victoria. "Cycling Fat." *Canadian Journal of Sports Science*; vol. 13, no. 4: 204-207.

Chapter 2: Lean Protein: a Metabolic Activator

1. Leaf, A., and Weber, P.C. "A New Era for Science in Nutrition." *The American Journal of Clinical Nutrition* (May 1987); supplement vol. 45, no. 5: 1048-1053.

2. Guyton, Arthur C. *Textbook of Medical Physiology.* 8th edition. W.B. Saunders Co.: 1991. p. 794. Lemon, P., *et. al.* "Effect of Initial Muscle Glycogen Levels on Protein Catabolism during Exercise." S Applied Physiology (1980); vol. 4: 624-629.

3. Carlson, L. "Report Fowls Up Egg-Cholesterol Debate." *The Physician and Sportsmedicine* (June 1991); vol. 19, no. 6: 17.

4. "What's Good For the Heart Is Good for the Colon." *Prevention* (July 1991): 22.

5. Raymond, N.G., Dwyer, S.T., Nevin, S.P., Kurtin, P. "An Approach to Protein Restriction in Children with Renal Insufficiency." *Pedriatic Nephrology* (1990); vol. 4: 145-151.

Chapter 3: Carbohydrates: Fuel and Fiber

1. *American Journal of Clinical Nutrition*, 45: 1197-201.

2. Wargovich, M.J. "Diet and Human Cancer: Anticarcinogens in Our Foods." 19th Annual Texas Human Nutrition Conference. *Diet, Lifestyles, and Health* (February 1992), Texas A&M University.

3. Smith, C.T., and Gilbertson-Smith, J.A. reported in *The American Council of Applied Clinical Nutrition*.

4. Ibid.

5. Kleiner, S.M. "Fiber Facts: How to Fight Disease with a High-Fiber Diet." *The Physician and Sportsmedicine* (October 1990); vol. 18, no. 10: 19, 22.

6. Ibid.

Chapter 4: EFAs and MCTs: the Healthy Fats

1. Brush, M. *Premenstrual Tension Syndrome.* Great Britain: St. Thomas Hospital, p. 37.

2. An excellent review of the literature on MCTs as well as an in-depth discussion of its use in the body can be found in an unpublished paper by: Roberson, A., and Parrillo, J. "Medium Chain Triglycerides in Sports." Parrillo

Performance, 5143 Kennedy Avenue, Cincinnati, Ohio 45213.

3. Seaton, T. B., Welle, S.L., Warenko, M.K., and Campbell, R.G. "Thermic Effect of Medium and Long Chain Triglycerides in Man." *The American Journal of Clinical Nutrition* (1986); 44: 630-634.

4. Dias, V. "Effects of Feeding and Energy Balance in Adult Humans." *Metabolism* (1990); vol. 39: 887-891.

Chapter 7: Vitamins : Metabolic Catalysts

1. Crocetti, A.F., and Guthrie, H.A. "Eating Behavior and Associated Nutrient Quality of Diets." Anarem Systems Research Corporation. New York, New York.

2. Council for Responsible Nutrition. "Benefits of Nutritional Supplements: A Reference Resource for Health Professionals, Media, and Industry." Washington, DC: 26.

3. Council for Responsible Nutrition: 10.

4. Ibid.

5. Swope, M. *Green Leaves of Barley*. p. 24.

6. Foley, D. "Block Cancer the 'Beta' Way." *Prevention* (April 1985): 28-32

7. Roblin, A. "Clean Out Your Cholesterol." *Prevention* (October 1988): 28.

8. Vaughn, L. "B$_6$: A Spectrum of Healing." *Prevention* (June 1984): 30.

9. Fletcher, A.M. "Can C Cure Your Cholesterol Woes?" *Prevention* (May 1991): 112-113.

10. Klein, M.A., and Perlmutter, C. "Vitamin C Against Cancer." *Prevention* (March 1991): 62-64, 127-131.

11. Perlmutter, C., with Gardey, T. "Diet and Immunity: The New Frontier." *Prevention* (October 1989): 51-52.

12. Applegate, L. "Booster Club." *Runner's World* (June 1991): 29-30.

13. Ibid.

Chapter 8: Minerals and Other Amazing Nutrients

1. Allen, L.H. "Calcium Bioavailability and Absorption: A Review." *The American Journal of Clinical Nutrition* (April 1982); 35.

2. Danielson, D.L. "Strengthen Your Bones With Exercise." *Prevention* (July 1981): 109.

3. Pacelli, L.C. "To Fortify Bones Use Calcium and Exercise." *The Physician and Sportsmedicine* (November 1989); vol. 17, no. 11: 27-28.

4. Vaughn, L. "The Health Power of Magnesium: A Medical Update." *Prevention* (July 1985): 79-80, 107-110.

5. Meade, J. "New Discoveries in Mineral Nutrition." *Prevention* (February 1986): 29-30.

6. Scrimshaw, N.S. "Iron Deficiency." *Scientific American* (October 1991): 48-49.

7. Malesky, G. "Vitamins for Energy." *Prevention* (December 1983): 20-26.

8. Shils, M., and Young, V. *Modern Nutrition in Health and Disease.* 7th ed. Philadelphia: Lea Febiger, 1988.

9. Scrimshaw, N.S. "Iron Deficiency." *Scientific American* (October 1991): 48.

10. Nielson, F.H. "Boron – An Overlooked Element of Potential Nutritional Importance." *Nutrition Today* (January/February 1988); 4-7.

11. Cowen, R. "Chromium May Prevent Type II Diabetes Onset." *Science News*; vol. 137: 214.

12. Freeland-Graves, J.H. "Manganese: An Essential Nutrient for Humans." *Nutrition Today* (November/December 1988): 13-19.

13. Ibid.

14. Council for Responsible Nutrition. "Benefits of Nutritional Supplements: A Reference Source for Health Professionals, Media, and Industry." Washington, DC; 22.

15. Hanaki, Y., Satoru, S., Ozawa, T., Ohno, M. "Ratio of Low-Density Lipoprotein Cholesterol to Ubiquinone As a Coronary Risk Factor." *The New England Journal of Medicine* (September 12, 1991); vol. 325, no. 11: 814-815.

16. Bucci, L., interview on KLIF.

17. Lau, B.H.S, et al. "Effect of an Odor-Modified Garlic Preparation on Blood Lipids." *Nutrition Research* (1987); 7: 139-149.

Chapter 9: Fat-Burning/Health-Building Exercise

1. Fiatarone, M.A., Marks, E.C., Ryan, N.D., et al. "High-Intensity Strength Training in Nonagenarians: Effect on Skeletal Muscle." *Journal of the American Medical Association* (1990); vol. 263, no. 22: 3029-3034.

2. Ike R.W., Lampman, R.M., and Castor, W.C. "Arthritis and Aerobic

Exercise: A Review." *The Physician and Sportsmedicine* (February 1989); vol. 17, no. 2: 128-139.

3. Gauthier, M. "Can Exercise Reduce the Risk of Cancer?" *The Physician and Sportsmedicine* (October 1986); vol. 14, no. 10: 171.

4. White, J. "Men: Exercise Reduces Colon Cancer Risk." *The Physician and Sportsmedicine* (December 1991); vol. 119, no. 12: 52, 54.

5. Gauthier, M. "Can Exercise Reduce the Risk of Cancer?" *The Physician and Sportsmedicine* (October 1986); vol. 14, no. 10: 177.

6. Associated Press. "Cardiovascular Ills Claim More in Single Year than Four Wars." *Evansville Courier* (January 18, 1988): 10.

7. Whitehurst, M., Menendez, E. "Endurance Training in Older Women: Lipid and Lipoprotein Responses." *The Physician and Sportsmedicine* (June 1991); vol. 19, no. 6: 95-102.

8. Wood, D., Stefanick, M., et al. "Changes in Plasma Lipids and Lipoproteins in Overweight Men during Weight Loss through Dieting as Compared with Exercise. *The New England Journal Of Medicine* (November 1988); vol. 319, no. 18: 1173-1179.

9. "Resistive Training Reduces Coronary Risk Factors." *The Physician and Sportsmedicine* (August 1988); vol. 16, no. 8: 155.

10. Fackelmann, K.A. "Regular Exercise Cuts Diabetes Risk." *Science News*; vol. 140: 36.

11. Monahan, T. "Exercise and Depression: Swapping Sweat for Serenity?" *The Physician and Sportsmedicine* (September 1986); vol. 14, no. 9: 192, 194.

12. McCann, L., and Holmes, D.S. "Influence of Aerobic Exercise on Depression." *Journal of Personality and Social Psychology* (1984); vol. 46, no. 5: 1142-1147.

13. Tucker, L. "Effect of Weight Training on Self-Concept: A Profile of Those Influenced Most." *Research Quarterly for Exercise and Sport* (1983); vol. 54, no. 4: 389-397.

14. Nutter, J. "Physical Activity Increases Bone Density." *NSCA Journal* (1986); vol. 8, no. 3: 67-69.

15. Taylor, F. "Building Bones with Bodybuilding." *The Physician and Sportsmedicine* (March 1991); vol. 19, no. 3: 51.

16. Cowart, V.S. "Can Exercise Help Women with PMS?" *The Physician and Sportsmedicine* (April 1989); vol. 17, no. 4: 168-178.

17. Goss, F.L., Robertson, R.J., Spina, R.J., et al. "Energy Cost of Bench Stepping and Pumping Light Handweights in Trained Subjects." *Research Quarterly for Exercise and Sport* (1989); vol. 60, no. 4: 369-372.

18. Riddle, P.K. "Attitudes, Beliefs, Behavioral Intentions, and Behaviors of Women and Men Toward Regular Jogging." *Research Quarterly for Exercise and Sport* (1980); vol. 54, no. 4: 663-674.

19. Porcari, J., McCarron, R., Kline, G., et al. "Is Fast Walking an Adequate Aerobic Training Stimulus for 30- to 69-Year-Old Men and Women?" *The Physician and Sportsmedicine* (February 1987); vol. 15, no. 2: 119-129.

20. Lippert, J. "The Fizzle Phenomenon." *Health* (February 1987): 55-57, 60.

21. Dishman, R. "Exercise Compliance: A New View for Public Health." *The Physician and Sportsmedicine* (May 1986); vol. 14, no. 5: 127-145.

Chapter 10: Nutritional Needs of Exercisers and Athletes

1. Lemon, P.W. "Protein and Exercise: Update 1987." *Med Sci Sports Exerc* (1987); 19: S179-S190.

2. McCarthy, P. "How Much Protein Do Athletes Really Need?" *The Physician and Sportsmedicine* (May 1989); vol. 17, no. 5: 170-175.

3. Leibovitz, B. and Blechman, S. "Proteins and Performance Update: A Special Interview with Dr. Peter Lemon, Ph.D." *Muscular Development* (September 1991): 79.

4. Spencer, H., Kramer, L., and Osis, D. "Do Protein and Phosphorus Cause Calcium Loss?" *The Journal of Nutrition* (June 1988); vol. 118, no. 6: 657-659.

5. Ibid.

6. O'Toole, M., Iwane, H., Douglas, P.S., et al. "Iron Status in Ultraendurance Athletes." *The Physician and Sportsmedicine* (December 1989); vol. 17, no. 12: 90-102.

7. Evans, G. "Anabolic Effect of Chromium Picolinate in Male Subjects." (University of Minnesota).

8. Wesson, M., McNaughton, L., Davies, P., and Tristram, S. "Effects of Oral Administration of Aspartic Acid Salts on the Endurance Capacity of Trained Athletes." *Research Quarterly for Exercise and Sport* (1988);vol. 59, no. 3: 234-239.

9. Applegate, L. "Booster Club." *Runner's World* (June 1991): 29-30.

10. Swinney, T. "Liver: The Premium Energy Food." *Ironman* (November 1991): 52.

11. Jacobson, B.H. "Effect of Amino Acids on Growth Hormone Release." *The Physician and Sportsmedicine* (January 1990); vol. 18, no. 1: 68.

Chapter 11: Leaner and Fitter for a Lifetime

1. Kleiner, S. "Seafood and Your Heart." *The Physician and Sportsmedicine* (April 1990); vol. 18, no. 4: 19-20.

2. Shils, M., and Young, V. *Modern Nutrition in Health and Disease.* 7th ed. Philadelphia: Lea Febiger, 1988.

3. Ibid.

4. Colgan, M. "Nutrition and Fitness News: Antioxidant Cocktail Slows Aging." *Muscular Development* (March 1991); vol. 28, no. 3: 60-61.

5. Rammohan, M., and Juan, D. "Effects of a Low-Calorie, Low-Protein Diet on Nutritional Parameters, and Routine Values in Nonobese Young and Elderly Subjects." *Journal of the American College of Nutrition* (1989); vol. 8, no. 6: 545-553.

6. Kavanaugh, T., and Shephard, R. "Can Regular Sports Participation Slow the Aging Process? Data on Masters Athletes." *The Physician and Sportsmedicine* (June 1990); vol. 18, no. 6: 94-104.

7. Work, J. "Strength Training: A Bridge to Independence for the Elderly." *The Physician and Sportsmedicine* (November 1989); vol. 17, no. 11: 143-140.

8. Shepard, J.G., and Pacelli, L.C. "Why Your Patients Shouldn't Take Aging Lying Down." *The Physician and Sportsmedicine* (November 1990); vol. 18, no. 11: 83-90.

Questions and Answers About Lean Bodies

Does the metabolism slow down with age?

Not really. What changes with many older people is their exercise and eating habits. They exercise less and eat less, and the metabolism slows down as a result. By eating the proper foods, exercising, and gradually increasing calories, anyone – regardless of age – can have a healthy metabolism.

I gained weight the first week. Is this a bad sign?

People who start the program with slow metabolisms, usually due to a history of roller-coaster dieting, typically gain some weight the first week. An initial gain, however, is the first step toward building your metabolism. Once your body starts becoming reoriented toward processing food, you will burn significant amounts of bodyfat.

I'm in high school, and I have a weight problem. Yet every time I go on a diet, the other kids at school know about it because they see me eat "diet" food – and not much of it. They give me a hard time. How can the Lean Bodies program help me?

I can sympathize. With all the prepackaged diet foods and shakes you are supposed to eat on low-calorie diets, you might as well scream out to the world "LOOK AT ME! I'M ON A DIET."

To answer your question, let me tell you the story of a father and son who went through the Lean Bodies program. The father is a physician, a urologist to be exact, and he and his 15-year-old-son have always loved to eat. But they got overweight as a result. After about six weeks on the program, they were close to shedding all the bodyfat they wanted to lose. That in itself is a success story – but the real point of this story is that the son was able to eat so much food, none of it pre-packaged diet food, that no one at school knew he was "dieting." That is what he liked about it. Also, I encourage young people on Lean Bodies to deviate a little more from the program, so they have even less peer pressure from friends.

The Lean Bodies program will work for you, and none of your friends will know you are on it. In fact, they will be surprised at all the food you get to eat. And they will probably be envious of how great you look after you have been on it.

I'm not used to eating breakfast, so I'm wondering how I'll get all my calories in?

Your question brings to mind John R., who was not a breakfast eater until he started the Lean Bodies program. But now, every morning, John eats four scrambled egg whites, two cups of brown rice, and two cups of oatmeal – a very hefty breakfast! Plus, John has lost 10 pounds and the roll around his middle.

Many people who go on the Lean Bodies program are not accustomed to eating breakfast. But once their metabolisms become more efficient at using food, they cannot wait to eat in the morning. In fact, they are ravenous! I predict the same thing will happen to you.

Are commercially frozen egg whites, such as those in the grocer's freezer, allowed on the Lean Bodies program?

No. These products do not have the nutrient value of real egg whites. Additionally, they contain chemical additives. The only time you should eat these products is when you are traveling and cannot get real egg whites.

Can I eat lamb or pork on the Lean Bodies program?

You should avoid these foods for the first seven weeks. Both are high in saturated fat.

Can I eat non-fat frozen yogurt?

Yes, but only after the first seven weeks. Afterwards, you may eat it occasionally.

If I eliminate bananas, how will I get my dietary potassium?

You will get this vital mineral from potatoes (a starchy carbohydrate), which contain at least as much potassium as bananas.

Is oat bran allowed on the Lean Bodies program?

Oatmeal is preferable to oat bran. As a pure fiber, oat bran has fewer carbohydrates than oatmeal. This means you will have less energy if you eat only oat bran. Oat bran, however, has been shown in studies to reduce LDL cholesterol. I suggest that you mix some oat bran in with your oatmeal.

I'm not really fond of oatmeal. What should I eat for breakfast?

You definitely do not have to eat oatmeal. There are many choices of whole grains on the program to choose for breakfast, including kashi, barley, corn grits, and shredded wheat.

Are there any fast foods I can eat on the Lean Bodies program?

Many fast food restaurants have salad bars, grilled chicken, and baked fish – so you can eat in these establishments and still stick to Lean Bodies fare.

For milk, can we drink soy milks?

Yes – as long as the product does not contain any simple sugars.

Regarding the mock meals, can I eat them more than twice a day?

Definitely, especially if you are hungry or low on energy.

Are sweeteners allowed on the Lean Bodies program?

The metabolism and use of sweeteners by the body are not well understood. For that reason, I suggest that you either avoid them or use them in moderation.

You recommend that we drink eight to 10 large glasses of water daily on the program. Can I replace some of that water with diet soft drinks?

Consider this: More than 70 percent of an eight-ounce glass of water is absorbed by the stomach, and only 15 to 20 percent of the same amount of soda is absorbed. Plus, diet soft drinks contain artificial sweeteners and other chemicals. How these additives are used by the body is unclear.

Look at it this way. Would you wash your clothes in soda pop? Then why clean your body that way? Remember – water is the universal solvent.

How much water should I drink each day?

Eight to 10 large glasses a day, especially if you are active.

Can I drink alcohol on the Lean Bodies program?

Alcohol has a dehydrating effect on the body; in other words, it upsets your body's water balance. Alcohol is also full of simple sugars, which are converted easily into bodyfat. Additionally, research has shown that moderate drinking can elevate blood pressure. I recommend that you stay away from alcohol until you have reached your bodyfat percentage goal. Then you may use it on a limited basis.

If omega-3s are such important nutrients, shouldn't I take omega-3 supplements?

As long as you include cold water, ocean-going, boney fish in your meal plans, you will get enough of the omega-3 fatty acids. In fact, just three ounces of fish a day supplies an ample amount of this pro-tective nutrient.

I've heard that vitamins begin to degrade in nutrient value the minute the bottle is opened. Is this true?

It depends on how you store your vitamins. Vitamins are a food, and like foods, they are subject to spoilage. Store your vitamins carefully and always keep their lids on tight.

How many lipotropic supplements should I take each day?

If you decide to add these supplements to the Lean Bodies program, take two lipotropics at breakfast and two more with dinner. Always check with your doctor first before taking any supplements.

What about sodium? How much – if any – should I take in?

Sodium or salt is a very controversial subject. To begin with, it is important to understand that sodium is an important mineral found in our bones, in the fluids surrounding our cells, and in the cardiovascular system. Sodium works together with potassium to assist nerve stimulation and regulate water balance. It is also involved in carbohydrate absorption.

The average person requires a minimum of one-tenth of a teaspoon of salt a day. An athlete who sweats profusely needs more – about a teaspoon a day.

Cooking with minimal amounts of salt does not cause problems, nor does eating fresh foods high in natural salt such as fish, carrots, beets, and poultry. Eating processed and junk foods, however, does lead to high, potentially dangerous levels of sodium intake.

The Lean Bodies program provides a healthy ratio of potassium to sodium: at least 2-to-1.

Is there any way to break the laxative habit?

There are three ways: Exercise, include plenty of fiber in your diet, and drink eight to 10 large glasses of water a day.

Isn't distilled water a purified form of water and therefore more healthy?

Not at all. Distilled water does not contain any minerals. By drinking distilled water, you run the risk of developing mineral deficiencies.

What does "enriched" mean?

Enriching is the replacement of nutrients in food which have been previously lost due to processing. The biggest problem with enriched foods is that only a few nutrients are added back in. Additionally, those replacement nutrients are synthetic and therefore not of the same nutritional value as those originally found in the food.

What are the desirable ranges for HDL cholesterol?

HDL cholesterol is the "good" cholesterol. A desirable range for a man is 45 and higher; for a woman, 50 to 55 or higher.

When is the best time to take my essential fatty acids?

You should take them with your meals.

Can I cook with safflower oil or any of the essential fatty acids allowed on the program?

Cooking causes oxidation – or breakdown – of the nutrients in the fats. For that reason, do not heat or cook the fats.

Is olive oil a source of essential fatty acids?

Olive oil is a monounsaturated fat. Although it has been touted as a "good fat," olive oil is not high in EFAs. To get your EFAs, stick to safflower oil, canola oil, and the other recommended oils.

With the amount of fat Americans eat, why are we so fat-deficient?

Americans do not have the right type of fat in their diets. The typical American diet is high in saturated fats, which contribute to cardiovascular disease, and low in essential fatty acids.

Does MCT oil have any calories?

Yes, approximately 114 calories per tablespoon.

If I take MCT oil, won't I gain fat?

No. MCT oil is burned so rapidly for energy that it is difficult for the body to store it as fat.

Can I use MCT oil in place of other fats?

No, MCT oil should be taken in addition to such fats as flaxseed oil, safflower oil, and canola oil. The reason is, MCT oil does not supply essential fatty acids.

How should I eat when under stress?

Proper nutrition during stressful times does much to minimize the stress. The first health habit that seems to be discarded during stress, however, is good nutrition. Many people either stop eating or start overeating. Both aggravate stress. When under stress, preserve your healthy eating habits. Proper nutrition is one of the best forms of stress management.

You emphasize animal protein on the Lean Bodies program, yet I'm a vegetarian. Can I follow the program?

It depends on what kind of vegetarian you are, and there are several. "Lacto-ovo-vegetarians," for example, limit their animal protein to dairy products and eggs. They can follow the program by using egg whites as their sole protein source, although this limits the variety of their food choices. "Semi-vegetarians," who avoid red meat but eat fish or chicken, can easily follow the program. "Vegans" avoid all animal proteins and therefore are not good candidates for the program.

Is low blood sugar correctable?

Yes. Ninety-five percent (95%) of all low blood sugar (hypoglycemia) is reactive, meaning that it is caused by factors within our control, such as diet. The other 5 percent of hypoglycemia is caused by medical problems such as pancreatic tumors.

Can proper nutrition boost the immune system?

Yes, especially when you supplement your diet with nutrients called antioxidants. These include vitamins A, C, E, betacarotene, selenium, and garlic.

I carry bodyfat mostly on my thighs and hips. How can I get rid of it?

By following the Lean Bodies program, you will shed bodyfat from all over your body – not just from specific areas. While you are losing, it is a good idea to try weight training, especially for those areas that seem flabbier than others. Even though you cannot spot reduce, you can spot tone.

I've noticed that I've gotten a little firmer since following the program. This has never happened to me on other diets. Before, my skin would always look loose. Can you explain this?

First of all, you are losing bodyfat, and this gives you more muscular definition. Second, you are taking bodyfat off gradually. This is important because low-calorie crash diets can damage the elasticity of your skin – especially if you go on and off them. Third, you are eating enough protein, which improves skin tone and elasticity. Also, regular weight training makes you firmer too.

I've heard that distribution of bodyfat is a risk factor for disease. Is this true?

Yes. Individuals who carry a lot of bodyfat around their waist are at risk for cardiovascular disease and diabetes.

Do I have to exercise to lose bodyfat on the Lean Bodies program?

No. In fact, I had one woman who lost 40 pounds on the program – without exercise. Exercise, however, is an important component of a healthy lifestyle – for many reasons. It helps accelerate the metabolism, makes the body run more efficiently, improves appearance, and lowers the risk factor for many deadly illnesses, among many other benefits.

The gym where I work out has recumbent stationary bicycles. Are these as effective as other stationary bicycles?

Recumbent bikes are designed so that you sit in an almost-supine position, close to the ground, with your legs stretched out in front of you. Research shows that the aerobic benefit of working out on recumbent bicycles is comparable to that of standard bicycles. Recumbent bikes are comfortable and easy to use.

I have increased my workouts from three times a week to five. Should I increase my calories?

Definitely. Anytime you increase exercise, you must increase calories.

I have a very busy schedule, and it is impossible to exercise. What should I do?

Try to schedule exercise in your week just like you would any other important appointment. Also, set short-term, performance-related goals. For example, pledge to work out just twice this week for a total of 20 minutes each time. Next week, increase your pledge to three times a week for 30 minutes each time. Make sure exercise is convenient and fun.

I travel out of town on business a lot, and I find that it is difficult to maintain my exercise program. What should I do?

First of all, it is important to plan ahead. Today, many hotels have on-site health clubs where guests can exercise – so you will want to make reservations at a place that has such a facility. Other hotels may have agreements with nearby gyms that allow hotel guests to work out for free or for a small charge.

If you are unsuccessful in locating a hotel with these services, invest in some easy-to-pack exercise gear, such as water-inflatable dumbbells or a jump rope. Or pack one of your favorite audio aerobics tapes, along with a tape recorder, so you can do some in-room exercise.

While out of town, try to walk as much as you can, and take the stairs instead of the elevator. This will help maintain your aerobic conditioning.

Lean Bodies Cooking

Egg White Scramble

6 egg whites, beaten

Spray a medium skillet with non-stick cooking spray. Add eggs and cook over low heat. Stir frequently until egg whites are set but still soft and moist. Serves 2.
(Serving = 1 lean protein)

You can vary the taste of scrambled egg whites by adding other ingredients such as green chiles, green peppers, onions, pimientos, and mushrooms. Try seasoning your egg whites with chili powder, dry mustard, thyme, and minced onion.

Potato Deviled Eggs

6 eggs, hard-boiled
2 medium baked potatoes, skin removed and mashed
1 tbsp. tarragon vinegar
1 tsp. mustard
1 tsp. freeze dried chives
⅛ tsp. turmeric

Cut eggs in half, lengthwise. Remove and discard yolks. Combine remaining ingredients and mix well. Fill egg white halves with the potato mixture. Chill before serving. Serves 2.
(Serving = 1 lean protein, 1 starchy carbohydrate)

Egg White Casserole

1½ cups cooked and thinly sliced potatoes
½ cup chopped green onion
1½ cups frozen peas, cooked
1 8-oz. can tomato sauce
¼ tsp. marjoram
½ tsp. chervil
6 egg whites
paprika for garnish

Preheat oven to 350 degrees. Spray a shallow 1½ quart baking dish with non-stick cooking spray. Arrange potato slices, onion, and peas in the dish. Combine tomato sauce, marjoram, and chervil. Pour mixture over peas.

Make 6 impressions in the mixture, and place egg whites in the impressions. Discard the yolks. Sprinkle casserole with paprika. Bake at 350 degrees for 25-30 minutes until eggs are set. Serves 2.

Note: This casserole may be prepared ahead of time. Simply cover and refrigerate several hours or overnight.
(Serving = 1 lean protein, 2 starchy carbohydrates)

Mexican Fish Fillets

1 lb. white fish fillets, fresh or frozen (thawed)
¼ cup vegetable juice
1 tbsp. finely chopped fresh cilantro
¼ tsp. garlic salt
2 tbsp. lemon juice

Arrange fish on an ungreased 8" x 8" x 2" baking dish. Combine vegetable juice, cilantro, garlic salt, and lemon juice, and pour over fish. Cover and bake at 350 degrees for 15 minutes. Uncover and bake until fish fillets flake easily with a fork (10-15 minutes). Serve with Jalapeno Tomato Sauce. Serves 4.

(Serving = 1 lean protein; ¼ lean, fibrous vegetable)

Jalapeno Tomato Sauce

1 cup chopped tomatoes
⅓ cup chopped onion
1 finely chopped jalapeno chili
¼ tsp. salt
½ tsp. oregano
1 tsp. parsley
2 cloves garlic, pressed
1 tbsp. lime juice

Combine all ingredients in a small, microwaveable dish. Heat on high for 1 to 2 minutes until hot.

Seasoned Fish Fillets with Spinach

1 lb. white fish fillets, fresh or frozen (thawed)
1 10-oz. pkg. frozen spinach, thawed
½ cup thinly sliced onion
¼ tsp. garlic salt
⅛ tsp. black pepper
¼ tsp. dry mustard
½ tsp. marjoram
½ cup chicken broth, defatted

1 tbsp. lemon juice

1 tbsp. cornstarch

¼ cup water

Arrange fish in a single layer in a 10-inch skillet. Spoon spinach over fillets. Arrange onion slices over fish and spinach. Combine garlic salt, pepper, dry mustard, marjoram, chicken broth, and lemon juice. Pour over fish. Bring to a boil. Then reduce heat, cover, and simmer until fish flakes easily with a fork (8 to 12 minutes). Remove fish to a platter and keep warm. Mix cornstarch and water. Stir into pan juices. Heat and stir until sauce is thickened and bubbly. Pour sauce over fish. Serve immediately. Serves 4.

(Serving = 1 lean protein; ½ lean, fibrous vegetable)

Cajun-Style Fish

1 lb. white fish fillets, fresh or frozen (thawed)

½ tsp. black pepper

½ tsp. cayenne pepper

½ tsp. white pepper

1 tsp. paprika

½ tsp. garlic salt

⅛ tsp. cumin

¼ tsp. marjoram

½ tsp. parsley flakes

2 tbsp. safflower oil

Combine all spices in a small bowl. Heat a thick-bottomed skillet over high heat. Brush fillets with oil and sprinkle with seasonings. Place in the skillet and cook 2 to 3 minutes on each side. Serves 4.

(Serving = 1 lean protein)

Barbecued Shrimp

1 lb. large shrimp, peeled and deveined
1 tbsp. low-salt soy sauce
2 tbsp. tomato paste
1 tbsp. red wine vinegar
1 tbsp. lemon juice
½ tsp. onion salt
½ tsp. garlic powder
1 tsp. barbecue seasoning
¼ tsp. cayenne pepper
¼ tsp. black pepper
1 tsp. oregano leaves

Place shrimp in a medium dish. Combine remaining ingredients and pour over shrimp. Cover and refrigerate several hours in a baking dish. Bake at 350 degrees until shrimp are thoroughly cooked (15 to 20 minutes). Serves 4.

(Serving = 1 lean protein)

Shrimp Scampi

1 lb. shrimp, peeled and deveined
3 cloves garlic, pressed
2 tbsp. safflower oil
2 tbsp. lemon juice
1 tbsp. tarragon vinegar
1 tbsp. low-salt soy sauce
¼ tsp. garlic powder
¼ tsp. black pepper
½ tsp. salt

Place shrimp in a medium dish. Combine garlic and oil. Pour over shrimp and marinate in the refrigerator for 30 minutes. Then, remove shrimp and marinade to a medium skillet. Combine the remaining ingredients and add to skillet. Saute mixture until shrimp are thoroughly cooked (5 minutes). Serves 4.

(Serving = 1 lean protein)

Tuna Oriental

1 cup sliced celery
½ cup chopped onion
1 cup chicken broth, defatted
one 7-oz. can water-packed albacore tuna, drained
one 4-oz. can mushrooms, drained
one 16-oz. can bean sprouts, drained
1 tbsp. low-salt soy sauce
one 6-oz. pkg. frozen snowpeas
1 tbsp. cornstarch
2 tbsp. water

In a medium skillet, saute celery and onion in broth until tender. Add tuna, mushrooms, bean sprouts, soy sauce, and snowpeas. Cover and simmer 8 to 10 minutes until snowpeas are tender. Mix cornstarch in water and add to skillet mixture. Stir and heat till thickened. Serves 4.

(Serving = 1 lean protein; 1 lean, fibrous vegetable)

Shrimp Salad

1 lb. medium cooked shrimp, shelled and deveined
1 cup chopped celery

½ cup chopped tomatoes

½ cup chopped onion

2 tbsp. chopped dill pickle

¼ tsp. salt

3 egg whites, hard-boiled and chopped

salad greens

Lean Thousand Island Dressing

Combine shrimp with celery, tomatoes, onions, dill pickle, salt, and egg whites. Add salad dressing and toss. Chill and serve over salad greens. Serves 4.

(Serving = 1 lean protein; ½ lean, fibrous vegetable)

Lean Thousand Island Dressing

½ cup non-fat yogurt

1 tbsp. tomato paste

1 tbsp. vegetable flakes

½ tsp. instant minced onion

¼ tsp. garlic powder

⅛ tsp. black pepper

Combine all ingredients. Chill several hours before serving. Makes ½ cup.

Fancy Tuna Salad

¼ cup non-fat yogurt

2 tbsp. white wine vinegar

2 tbsp. chicken broth, defatted

1 tsp. minced onion

1 tsp. parsley flakes

½ tsp. lemon peel

⅛ tsp. black pepper

1 tsp. vegetable flakes

two 7-oz. cans water-packed albacore tuna, drained

1 cup alfalfa sprouts

2 cups asparagus, cooked

1 cup tomatoes, wedge cut

3 egg whites, hard-boiled and chopped

Combine the first 8 ingredients to make a dressing and chill while preparing the rest of the salad. Combine tuna and alfalfa sprouts. Arrange tuna in the center of four salad plates. Surround with asparagus and tomatoes. Pour the chilled dressing over the salad. Garnish with chopped egg whites. Serves 4.

(Serving = 1 lean protein; 1 lean, fibrous vegetable)

Smothered Chicken

2 whole chicken breasts, split and skinned

1 cup sliced onion

1 clove garlic, pressed

one 14½-oz. can stewed tomatoes

2 tsp. parsley flakes

½ tsp. seasoned salt

½ tsp. basil

¼ tsp. marjoram

¼ cup chicken broth, defatted

one 4-oz. can mushrooms, drained

1 tbsp. cornstarch dissolved in 2 tbsp. water

Arrange chicken breasts in a large microwaveable casserole dish. Combine remaining ingredients to make a sauce and pour over chicken. Cover with wax paper and microwave on high for 8 minutes. Stir and rotate dish ½ turn. Heat 8 to 10 minutes until chicken is thoroughly cooked. Remove wax paper and let stand 5 minutes before serving. Serves 4.

(Serving = 1 lean protein; ½ lean, fibrous vegetable)

Turkey Chili

1 ¼ lbs. ground turkey breast, skin removed

1 tbsp. safflower oil

one 8-oz. can tomato sauce

2 cups water

one 14-oz. can tomatoes

2 tsp. minced onion

½ tsp. garlic powder

1 ½ tsp. paprika

1 tbsp. cumin

1 tsp. ground oregano

1 tsp. salt

2 tsp. cayenne pepper

2 - 3 tbsp. chili powder (to taste)

1 cup uncooked kidney beans, soaked overnight and drained

In a large saucepan, brown turkey in oil. Add remaining ingredients and simmer 1 to 2 hours until beans are tender. Serves 4.

(Serving = 1 lean protein; 1 starchy carbohydrate; ½ lean, fibrous vegetable)

Spicy Meat Loaf

1 ¼ lbs. ground turkey breast, skin removed

½ cup old-fashioned oats

one 8-oz. can tomato sauce

½ cup vegetable juice

1 egg white

1 tsp. red wine vinegar

1 tsp. chili powder

½ tsp. salt

1 clove garlic, pressed

1 tbsp. safflower oil

½ cup finely chopped onion

½ cup finely chopped celery

Combine the first 8 ingredients and mix well. Saute onion, celery, and garlic in oil until onions are transparent. Add to turkey mixture. Mix well. Shape into a loaf and press into an 8" x 4" loaf pan. Bake 1 hour at 350 degrees. Serves 4.

(Serving = 1 lean protein)

Savory Poultry Strips

3 cups cooked chicken or turkey breasts, cut into strips

2 cups broccoli florets

1 cup freeze-dried mushrooms

½ cup chopped green onion

2 tbsp. low-salt soy sauce

2 tsp. grated fresh ginger root

1 tsp. summer savory

2 tsp. lemon juice

2 cups chicken broth, defatted

2 tbsp. cornstarch dissolved in ¼ cup water

Combine all ingredients, except the cornstarch mixture, in a large skillet. Bring to a boil. Reduce heat, cover, and simmer 15 minutes until broccoli is tender. Add cornstarch mixture. Heat and stir until thickened. Serves 4.

(Serving = 1 lean protein; ½ lean, fibrous vegetable)

South-of-the-Border Salad

1 lb. ground turkey breast, skin removed

1 clove garlic, pressed

¼ cup chopped onion

½ cup water

½ tsp. Kitchen Bouquet

¼ cup tomato paste mixed with ¾ cup water

¼ tsp. ground oregano

1 tbsp. chili powder

¾ tsp. cumin

1 tsp. paprika

¼ tsp. cayenne pepper

8 cups lettuce

1 cup tomato, wedge cut

1 ½ cup cooked kidney beans

¼ cup chopped green onion

⅓ cup Vegetable French Dressing

1 recipe Spicy Salsa

Brown turkey, garlic, and onion in water and Kitchen Bouquet. Stir frequently to keep turkey crumbly. Combine tomato paste mixture, oregano, chili powder, cumin, paprika, and cayenne pepper. Add to turkey. Simmer 10 to 15 minutes until mixture is thickened. Combine lettuce, tomatoes, kidney beans, and green onions. At serving time, mix salad, turkey, and Vegetable French Dressing. Toss. Serve with Spicy Salsa. Serves 4.

(Serving = 1 lean protein; ½ starchy carbohydrate; 1 lean, fibrous vegetable)

Vegetable French Dressing

½ cup cider vinegar

½ cup vegetable juice

2 tbsp. lemon juice

¼ cup chopped cucumber

2 tsp. vegetable flakes

½ tsp. celery flakes

½ tsp. garlic powder

⅛ tsp. black pepper

Combine all ingredients in a blender. Blend until well mixed. Chill several hours before serving. Makes 1½ cups.

Spicy Salsa

1 cup finely chopped tomatoes

½ cup finely chopped onion

1 tbsp. finely chopped green chilies

1 finely chopped jalapeno pepper

¼ cup vegetable juice

½ tsp. herb seasoning

¼ tsp. salt (optional)

Combine all ingredients in a jar. Chill for 1 hour before serving. Makes 1¼ cups.

Chicken Broth

8 cups water
1 to 3 lbs. chicken parts (wings, backs, necks, and ribs)
1 onion, cut into wedges
2 stalks celery, cut into chunks
1 carrot, cut into chunks
1 tsp. parsley flakes
1 bay leaf
¼ tsp. black pepper

Combine all ingredients in a stock pot. Bring to a boil. Reduce heat, cover, and simmer for 2 to 3 hours until chicken is very tender. Remove bones and strain broth. Cover broth and refrigerate until fat congeals on top. Skim off fat and discard. Strain broth through several thicknesses of cheesecloth to remove any remaining fat. Refrigerate or freeze broth. Makes 8 cups.

Note: Freeze some broth in ice cube trays that measure 2 tablespoons. When frozen, these broth cubes can be stored in a freezer bag and used when recipes call for small amounts of chicken broth.

Chicken and Rice Soup

1 cup uncooked brown rice
4 cups chicken broth, defatted

4 cups water

1 cup chopped onion

one 28-oz. can chopped tomatoes

one 4-oz. can green chilies

3 cups chicken, cooked and skinned

½ tsp. garlic salt

1 tbsp. chili powder

2 tsp. cumin

2 tsp. cilantro

¼ tsp. black pepper

2 tbsp. lime juice

¼ cup chopped green onion, for garnish

½ cup chopped tomatoes, for garnish

Combine brown rice, broth, water, and onions in a large stock pot. Bring to a boil. Reduce heat, cover, and simmer 45 minutes. Add all ingredients, except green onions and tomatoes. Cover and simmer 30 to 45 minutes until rice is tender. Garnish with green onions and tomatoes. Serves 4.

(Serving = 1 lean protein; 1 starchy carbohydrate; ½ lean, fibrous vegetable)

Potato Soup with Chicken

6 cups chicken broth, defatted

1½ cups cooked and shredded chicken breast

1 cup chopped onion

2 cups diced potatoes

1 cup frozen peas

one 10-oz pkg. fresh spinach

½ cup chopped fresh parsley

1 tbsp. vegetable flakes

½ tsp. garlic salt

¼ tsp. white pepper

¼ tsp. lemon peel

Combine all ingredients in a large stock pot. Bring to a boil. Reduce heat, cover, and simmer 45 to 55 minutes until tender. Serves 4. (Serving = ½ lean protein; 1 starchy carbohydrate; ½ lean, fibrous vegetable)

Turkey and Vegetable Bisque

1 lb. pinto beans, soaked overnight and drained

6 cups water

2 cups vegetable juice

2 cups chicken broth, defatted

2 bay leaves

2 lbs. ground turkey breast, skin removed

1 cup chopped onion

2 cloves garlic, minced

1 cup sliced green pepper

1 cup sliced celery

1 cup sliced carrots

one 14-oz. can chopped tomatoes

1 tsp. black pepper

1 tsp. cayenne pepper

½ tsp. cumin

½ tsp. ground ginger

1 tbsp. vegetable flakes

2 tsp. herb seasoning

1 tsp. hickory salt

1 tsp. liquid smoke

Combine drained beans, water, broth, vegetable juice, and bay leaf in a large stock pot. Bring to a boil for 10 minutes. Reduce heat, cover, and simmer 1 hour. Brown turkey breast in a medium skillet sprayed with non-stick spray. Add browned turkey and remaining ingredients, cover, and simmer 45 to 55 minutes until tender. Serves 8. (Serving = 1 lean protein; 1 starchy carbohydrate; ½ lean, fibrous vegetable)

Southern Salad

3 cups black-eyed peas, cooked

1 cup chopped tomatoes

⅓ cup chopped green onion

2 tbsp. chopped green chilies

1 tsp. chopped jalapeno pepper

¼ cup non-fat yogurt

½ tsp. marjoram

1 tsp. celery flakes

2 tbsp. rice wine vinegar

¼ tsp. garlic powder

⅛ tsp. black pepper

Combine black-eyed peas, tomatoes, green onion, green chilies, and jalapeno pepper in a bowl. Mix remaining ingredients, pour over vegetables, and toss. Chill several hours before serving. Serves 4. (Serving = 1 starchy carbohydrate; ¼ lean, fibrous vegetable)

Potato and Green Bean Salad

3 cups cooked and cubed potatoes

3 cups green beans, cooked

¼ cup non-fat yogurt

1 tbsp. celery flakes

1 tbsp. white wine vinegar

¼ tsp. garlic salt

1 tsp. instant minced onion

⅛ tsp. black pepper

Combine potatoes and green beans in a bowl. Mix remaining ingredients together. Pour over vegetables and toss. Chill several hours before serving. Serves 4.

(Serving = 1 starchy carbohydrate; 1 lean, fibrous vegetable)

Potato Salad Vinaigrette

3 cups potatoes

½ cup sliced red onion, separated into rings

1 cup sliced celery

½ cup sliced radishes

1 tsp. vegetable flakes

½ tsp. Italian seasoning

⅓ cup Spicy Vinaigrette

Cook potatoes in boiling water until near tender. Drain and cool. Cut potatoes into cubes. Combine all ingredients and toss gently with Spicy Vinaigrette to coat. Chill several hours before serving. Serves 4.

(Serving = 1 starchy carbohydrate; ½ lean, fibrous vegetable)

Spicy Vinaigrette

⅔ *cup cider vinegar*

⅓ *cup chicken broth, defatted*

1½ tsp. dry mustard

1 tsp. basil

1 tsp. oregano leaves

1 tsp. paprika

¼ tsp. garlic powder

¼ tsp. cayenne pepper

Combine all ingredients in a small, covered jar. Shake well. Refrigerate and use as needed. Makes 1 cup.

Rice and Vegetable Chowder

1 cup uncooked brown rice

4 cups chicken broth, defatted

one 28-oz. cans of tomatoes, chopped

two 6-oz. cans of tomato paste

6 cups water

1 cup chopped onion

1 bay leaf

½ tsp. garlic powder

2 tsp. herb seasoning

½ tsp. seasoned salt

¼ tsp. black pepper

1 tsp. basil

1 tsp. paprika

3 cups shredded cabbage

1 cup sliced carrots

2 cups sliced celery

1 cup chopped green pepper

one 4-oz. can chopped green chilies

Combine the first 12 ingredients in a large stock pot. Bring to a boil. Reduce heat, cover, and simmer 45 minutes. Add remaining ingredients and bring to a boil. Reduce heat, cover, and simmer for 30 to 45 minutes until all ingredients are tender. Discard bay leaf. Serves 8. (Serving = ½ starchy carbohydrate; 1 lean, fibrous vegetable)

Navy Bean Soup and Vegetables

1 lb. navy beans, soaked overnight and drained

2 qts. water

1 bay leaf

1 cup chopped onion

1 cup sliced carrots

1 cup sliced celery

one 8-oz. can tomato sauce

one 28-oz. can tomatoes

1 tsp. parsley flakes

1 tsp. summer savory

2 tsp. herb seasoning

¼ tsp. liquid smoke

2 tsp. vinegar

½ tsp. hickory salt

¼ cup chopped green onion, for garnish

1 cup chopped tomatoes, for garnish

Combine drained beans, water, and bay leaf in a large stock pot. Bring to a boil for 10 minutes. Reduce heat, cover, and simmer 1 hour. Add remaining ingredients, except green onions and tomatoes. Cover and simmer until beans are tender (2 to 3 hours). Add additional water if soup is too thick. Discard bay leaf. Garnish with green onions and tomatoes. Serves 8.

(Serving = 1 starchy carbohydrate; ½ lean, fibrous vegetable)

Split Pea Soup

1 lb. split peas

7 cups water

1 cup chopped onion

2 cups sliced celery

1 cup sliced carrots

1 bay leaf

1 tbsp. liquid smoke

1 tsp. hickory salt

1 tbsp. vegetable flakes

1 tsp. herb seasoning

½ tsp. marjoram

¼ tsp. white pepper

1 tsp. parsley flakes

½ tsp. garlic powder

¼ cup chopped green onion, for garnish

Combine all ingredients, except green onions, in a large stock pot. Bring to a boil. Reduce heat, cover, and simmer 1 to 2 hours until peas are very soft. Discard bay leaf. Serve garnished with green onions. Serves 6.

(Serving = 1 starchy carbohydrate; ¾ lean, fibrous vegetable)

Tomato and Corn Soup

5 cups tomatoes, cut into large chunks

2 cups chicken broth, defatted

1 ½ cups corn, frozen or fresh (kernels cut from cob)

½ cup water

1 tbsp. vegetable flakes

1 tsp. herb seasoning

½ tsp. summer savory

¼ tsp. basil

1 bay leaf

⅛ tsp. black pepper

1 tbsp. fresh parsley sprigs for garnish

Combine tomatoes and chicken broth in a medium saucepan. Bring to a boil. Reduce heat, cover, and simmer until tomatoes are very tender. Combine corn, water, vegetable flakes, herb seasoning, summer savory, basil, bay leaf, and black pepper in a large saucepan. Cook 8 to 10 minutes until corn is tender. Put cooked tomatoes through a sieve. Discard skin and seeds. Add liquid to the corn mixture. Cover and simmer soup 10 to 15 minutes to blend flavors. Discard the bay leaf. Serve garnished with fresh parsley. Serves 4.

(Serving = 1 starchy carbohydrate; 1 lean, fibrous vegetable)

Brown Rice Supreme

1 cup uncooked brown rice (or 3 cups cooked)

1 cup chicken broth, defatted

½ cup julienned carrots

½ cup julienned zucchini

½ tsp. garlic powder

½ tsp. grated lemon peel

1 tbsp. lemon juice

½ tsp. nutmeg

1 tbsp. grated ginger root

2 tbsp. chopped fresh parsley

Cook rice according to package instructions. Add remaining ingredients, except parsley, to the cooked rice. Simmer 6 to 10 minutes, stirring occasionally. Garnish with parsley. Serves 4.

(Serving = 1 starchy carbohydrate; 1 lean, fibrous vegetable)

Brown Rice and Mushrooms

1 cup uncooked brown rice (3 cups cooked)

1 cup chicken broth, defatted

½ cup sliced green onion

½ cup sliced celery

1 cup sliced fresh mushrooms

1 tbsp. low-salt soy sauce

1 tsp. summer savory

½ tsp. marjoram

Cook rice according to package instructions. Saute onions, celery, and mushrooms in broth in a medium skillet until tender. Add cooked rice and remaining ingredients. Simmer 6 to 10 minutes. Stir occasionally. Serves 4.

(Serving = 1 starchy carbohydrate; ¼ lean, fibrous vegetable)

Festive Corn

4 cups frozen corn
¼ cup chopped onion
¼ cup chopped green pepper
½ cup chopped tomatoes
¼ cup water
¼ tsp. seasoned salt

Combine all ingredients in a medium, microwaveable dish. Cover. Microwave on high until vegetables are tender (6 to 8 minutes). Stir once during heating. Serves 4.

(Serving = 1 starchy carbohydrate; ¼ lean, fibrous vegetable)

Sauteed New Potatoes

2 lbs. new potatoes
2 tbsp. safflower oil
¼ cup finely chopped green onion
2 tbsp. fresh parsley
½ tsp. garlic salt
½ tsp. herb seasoning
⅛ tsp. black pepper

Cook potatoes in boiling, salted water for 15 to 20 minutes until tender. Drain and cool. Cut potatoes into ¼-inch slices. Heat oil in a large, non-stick skillet. Add potatoes and sprinkle with green onions, parsley, garlic salt, herb seasoning, and pepper. Cook 4 to 5 minutes until potatoes start to brown. Continue cooking until golden brown. Serves 4.

(Serving = 1 starchy carbohydrate)

Minted Peas

3 cups frozen peas

¼ cup water

½ tsp. vegetable flakes

2 tsp. mint flakes

Combine all ingredients in a medium, microwaveable dish. Cover. Microwave on high until tender (about 6 to 8 minutes). Stir occasionally during heating. Serves 4.

(Serving = 1 starchy carbohydrate)

Hickory-Smoked Pinto Beans

1 lb. pinto beans

6 cups water

1 cup chopped onion

2 cloves garlic, pressed

one 14-oz. can tomatoes, chopped

¼ tsp. red pepper flakes

2 tsp. chili powder

2 tsp. herb seasoning

1 tsp. hickory salt

2 tsp. liquid smoke

1 tsp. onion powder

Wash beans and soak overnight covered in water. Drain. Combine drained beans and fresh water in a stock pot. Bring to a boil and boil for 10 minutes. Add remaining ingredients and reduce heat. Cover and simmer until beans are tender (1 to 2 hours). If beans need to be thickened, dissolve 2 tbsp. of cornstarch in ¼ cup water and add to

beans. Cook and stir until thickened. Serves 8.
(Serving = 1 starchy carbohydrate)

Oven-Fried Potatoes

2 lbs. potatoes
seasonings as desired (chili powder, garlic powder, onion powder,
    hickory salt, seasoned salt, paprika, or Italian seasoning)
non-stick spray

Scrub potatoes but do not peel. Boil potatoes until almost tender (15 to 20 minutes). Drain and refrigerate. When potatoes are cool, carefully peel them. Slice lengthwise into French fries or crosswise into cottage fries. Spread potatoes on a non-stick baking sheet sprayed with non-stick spray. Season as desired. Spray seasoned potatoes with non-stick spray. Brown in the oven at 450 degrees for 15 to 18 minutes. Turn and brown on the other side for 10 to 15 minutes. When done, potatoes should be crisp. Serves 6 to 8.
(Serving = 1 starchy carbohydrate)

Herbed Potato Skins

4 medium baking potatoes
herb seasoning
seasoned salt or garlic salt to taste

Scrub potatoes thoroughly and set aside to dry. Using a paring knife, peel ¾-inch wide strips of skin from the potatoes. Peel end to end. Remove a thin layer of potato pulp with each strip. Drop peeled potatoes into cold, salted water to cover and reserve for another use.

Place potato peels, skin side up, on a shallow baking pan that has been sprayed with non-stick spray. Bake at 450 degrees for 15 to 20 minutes until potato skins are crisp and golden. Sprinkle with seasonings. Potato skins may be made ahead of time, refrigerated or frozen, and then reheated at 450 degrees for 5 to 10 minutes. Serves 4. (Serving = 1 starchy carbohydrate)

Baked Potatoes with Tangy Toppers

4 medium baked potatoes

For parsley topping: Combine ½ cup non-fat yogurt, 1 tbsp. chopped fresh parsley, ½ tsp. onion powder, ¼ tsp. basil, and ⅛ black pepper. Spoon on baked potatoes. Serves 4.

For dill topping: Combine ½ cup non-fat yogurt, ½ tsp. mustard, ¼ tsp. dill weed, ½ tsp. onion powder, and ¼ tsp. garlic powder. Spoon on baked potatoes. Serves 4.

For chive topping: Combine ½ cup non-fat yogurt, 1 tbsp. chopped fresh parsley, 1 tbsp. fresh chopped chives, and ½ tsp. instant onion. Spoon on baked potatoes. Serves 4.
(Serving = 1 starchy carbohydrate)

Mashed Potatoes

2 lbs. potatoes
1 bay leaf
2 tsp. celery flakes
1 clove garlic
⅛ tsp. black pepper

1 tsp. arrowroot

¼ tsp. salt

1 tbsp. non-fat yogurt

Wash, peel, and quarter potatoes. Boil potatoes, bay leaf, celery flakes, and garlic until potatoes are tender. With a slotted spoon, transfer potatoes to a large bowl. Reserve potato water. Combine arrowroot with ¼ cup potato water and add to potatoes along with salt and pepper. Mash potatoes, adding more potato water if needed. Add yogurt and stir. Serves 4.

(Serving = 1 starchy carbohydrate)

Beans and Rice Creole

1 lb. red beans, soaked overnight and drained

3 cups chicken broth, defatted

3 cups water

2 bay leaves

1 tsp. paprika

1 tsp. oregano leaves

1 tsp. cayenne pepper

2 tsp. salt

2 tsp. chili powder

2 cups chopped onion

1 cup chopped green pepper

1 cup chopped celery

2 cloves garlic, minced

1 14-oz. can tomatoes

1 8-oz. can tomato sauce

1 tbsp. Worchestershire sauce

2 tbsp. parsley flakes

1 cup uncooked brown rice

Place drained beans in a large stock pot. Add broth, water, bay leaves, paprika, oregano, cayenne pepper, salt, and chili powder. Bring to a boil and boil for 10 minutes. Reduce heat and simmer 1 hour. Add remaining ingredients. Continue cooking 1 to 2 hours until beans and rice are tender and liquid is reduced. Serves 8.

(Serving = 2 starchy carbohydrates; 1 lean, fibrous vegetable)

Sweet Potatoes with Maple

2 lbs. sweet potatoes

½ tsp. cinnamon

¼ tsp. maple flavoring

⅛ tsp. rum extract

¼ cup hot water

Wash sweet potatoes and scrub thoroughly. Place in a stock pot of boiling water. Cover and boil until tender. Drain. When potatoes are cool enough to handle, peel and mash. Add cinnamon, maple flavoring, rum extract, and hot water. Continue beating until light and fluffy. Serves 4.

(Serving = 1 starchy carbohydrate)

Asparagus Salad Vinaigrette

4 cups asparagus spears, fresh or frozen

¼ cup water

2 tbsp. chopped pimientos

⅓ cup Tarragon Vinaigrette

Combine asparagus and water in a medium, microwaveable dish. Cover. Microwave on high until asparagus is just tender (6 minutes). Drain and chill. Add pimientos to the Tarragon Vinaigrette and pour over asparagus. Chill several hours. Serve over lettuce if desired. Serves 4.

(Serving = 1 lean, fibrous vegetable)

Tarragon Vinaigrette

½ cup tarragon vinegar

¼ cup chicken broth, defatted

2 tbsp. chopped pimientos

2 tbsp. chopped dill pickle

½ tsp. onion salt

2 tsp. parsley flakes

¼ tsp. black pepper

¼ tsp. lemon peel

Combine all ingredients in a small, covered jar. Shake well. Refrigerate and use as needed. Makes 1 cup.

Gala Cole Slaw

4 cups shredded cabbage

2 cups shredded carrots

¼ cup thinly sliced celery

¼ cup thinly sliced green onion

¼ cup non-fat yogurt

⅛ tsp. dry mustard

1 tsp. dill weed

1 tsp. vegetable flakes

⅛ tsp. onion salt

⅛ tsp. white pepper

½ tsp. caraway

Combine cabbage, carrots, celery, and green onion. Mix remaining ingredients together. Pour over vegetables and toss. Cover and chill several hours. Serves 4.

(Serving = 1 lean, fibrous vegetable)

Marinated Vegetable Salad

4 cups sliced cucumbers

1 cup sliced onion, separated into rings

1 cup tomatoes, wedge cut

1 ½ cups cider vinegar

½ cup water

½ tsp. marjoram

½ tsp. salt

⅜ tsp. black pepper

1 tsp. herb seasoning

Layer cucumbers and onions in a 2-quart bowl. Place tomatoes on top. Combine remaining ingredients and pour over vegetables. Refrigerate several hours or overnight. Stir once to ensure that all the vegetables marinate. Serves 6.

(Serving = 1 lean, fibrous vegetable)

Italian Salad

1 ½ cups green beans, fresh or frozen
¼ cup water
1 ½ cups sliced zucchini
1 cup sliced tomatoes
½ cup sliced onion, separated into rings
2 tbsp. chopped fresh parsley
½ cup Spicy Vinaigrette

Combine green beans and water in a medium, microwaveable dish. Cover and microwave until near tender (6 to 8 minutes). Drain. Add zucchini, tomatoes, onion, and parsley. Pour Italian Vinaigrette over salad and toss. Cover and chill several hours or overnight. Stir twice. Drain to serve. Serves 4.

(Serving = 1 lean, fibrous vegetable)

Caesar Salad

1 tbsp. safflower oil
1 clove garlic, pressed
8 cups Romaine lettuce (1 head)
1 egg (yolk to be discarded)
1 small lemon
1 tsp. paprika
½ tsp. salt
⅛ tsp. black pepper
¼ tsp. red wine vinegar
¼ tsp. dry mustard

Crush garlic and soak in oil. Let this stand while you prepare the salad. Wash lettuce, drain thoroughly, and tear into bite-sized pieces. Coddle egg in boiling water for 1 minute. Break egg and discard yolk. Add egg white to lettuce and toss. Cut lemon in half and thoroughly squeeze juice over salad. Toss. Add paprika, salt, pepper, red wine vinegar, dry mustard, and garlic and oil mixture. Toss thoroughly. Serves 4. (Serving = 1 lean, fibrous vegetable)

Spinach Vinaigrette Salad

½ tsp. grated orange peel
Lemon Mustard Vinaigrette
4 cups washed and torn spinach
4 cups washed and torn lettuce
1 cup sliced fresh mushrooms
¼ cup chopped pimientos
½ cup sliced red onion, separated into rings

Add orange peel to Lemon Mustard Vinaigrette and chill several hours. Combine spinach, lettuce, mushrooms, pimientos, and red onion in a large salad bowl. Shake salad dressing and pour over salad. Toss and serve immediately. Serves 4.
(Serving = 1 lean, fibrous vegetable)

Lemon Mustard Vinaigrette

½ cup red wine vinegar
¼ cup lemon juice
¼ cup chicken broth, defatted
½ tsp. garlic salt
2 tsp. parsley flakes

1 tsp. dry mustard

½ tsp. paprika

Combine all ingredients in a small, covered jar. Shake well. Refrigerate and use as needed. Makes 1 cup.

Onion Soup

6 onions, sliced thickly

2 tbsp. safflower oil

4 cups chicken broth, defatted

4 cups water

1 cup shredded carrots

1 cup shredded zucchini

3 bay leaves

3 whole cloves

1 tsp. herb seasoning

½ tsp. salt

¼ tsp. black pepper

¼ tsp. thyme

½ cup water

2 tbsp. cornstarch

Cook onions in oil in a stock pot for 20 to 30 minutes. Stir frequently until onions are lightly browned and glazed. Add all ingredients except ½ cup water and cornstarch. Bring to a boil. Reduce heat, cover, and simmer for 45 minutes. Mix water and cornstarch. Add to soup and cook until slightly thickened and bubbly. Serves 8.

(Serving = 1 lean, fibrous vegetable)

Tomato Soup

3 cups tomato juice
2 stalks celery, cut in chunks
2 slices onion
1 bay leaf
6 whole cloves
1 tsp. sliced ginger root
½ tsp. paprika
1 cup chicken broth, defatted
1 tsp. low-salt soy sauce
2 tbsp. chopped green onion
4 slices lemon

Combine tomato juice, celery, onion, bay leaf, cloves, ginger root, and paprika in a medium saucepan. Bring to a boil. Reduce heat, cover, and simmer for 20 minutes. Strain soup and discard seasonings. Return liquid to saucepan. Add chicken broth and soy sauce. Cook until hot. Garnish with lemon slices and green onion. Serves 4. (Serving = ½ lean, fibrous vegetable)

Asparagus Oriental

4 cups fresh asparagus
2 tbsp. minced onion
2 tbsp. water
1 tbsp. low-salt soy sauce
1 tsp. grated ginger root

Rinse asparagus and break off tough root ends. If asparagus spears are thick, cut crosswise into 1-inch pieces. Combine all ingredients in a medium microwaveable dish. Cover. Microwave on high until tender (8 to 10 minutes). Serves 4.

(Serving = 1 lean, fibrous vegetable)

Beets l'Orange

2 lbs. fresh beets
⅓ cup chicken broth, defatted
1 tbsp. cornstarch dissolved in 1 tbsp. water
1 tsp. grated orange peel
1 tsp. celery flakes
⅛ tsp. cinnamon

Place unpeeled beets in water in a large saucepan. Cook in boiling water until beets are tender (40 to 60 minutes). Drain, peel, and slice beets. Combine broth, dissolved cornstarch, orange peel, celery flakes, and cinnamon in a medium saucepan. Cook and stir until thickened. Add sliced beets and heat. Serves 4.

(Serving = 1 lean, fibrous vegetable)

Spicy Vegetables

2 cups broccoli florets, fresh or frozen
2 cups thinly sliced carrots
¼ cup sliced green onion
¾ cup chicken broth, defatted
¼ tsp. seasoned salt
¼ tsp. cayenne pepper
¼ tsp. lemon pepper
2 tbsp. non-fat yogurt

Combine all ingredients, except yogurt, in a medium, microwaveable dish. Cover. Microwave on high for 8 to 10 minutes. Stir occasionally during heating. Garnish with non-fat yogurt. Microwave on high for 1 minute. Serves 4.

(Serving = 1 lean, fibrous vegetable)

Broccoli Italiano

4 cups broccoli florets, fresh or frozen
one 14-oz. can tomatoes
⅛ tsp. garlic powder
¼ tsp. seasoned salt
1 tsp. Italian seasoning
⅛ tsp. black pepper

Combine all ingredients in a medium, microwaveable dish. Cover. Microwave on high for 8 to 10 minutes. Stir after 4 minutes. Serves 4.

(Serving = 1 lean, fibrous vegetable)

Caraway Cabbage

6 cups shredded cabbage
⅓ cup chicken broth, defatted
½ tsp. salt
⅛ tsp. black pepper
1 tsp. caraway

Combine all ingredients in a medium, microwaveable dish. Cover. Microwave on high 8 to 10 minutes. Stir occasionally. Serves 4.

(Serving = 1 lean, fibrous vegetable)

Carrots with Ginger

1 lb. thinly sliced carrots

1 cup water

2 tsp. grated ginger root

½ tsp. cinnamon

½ tsp. orange peel

Combine all ingredients in a medium, microwaveable dish. Cover. Microwave on high until tender (10 to 12 minutes). Stir occasionally. Serves 4.

(Serving = 1 lean, fibrous vegetable)

Cauliflower with Toasted Oats

4 cups cauliflower florets, fresh or frozen

½ cup chicken broth, defatted

½ tsp. salt

¼ tsp. dry mustard

2 hard boiled egg whites, chopped

2 tbsp. chopped fresh parsley

3 tbsp. toasted oats

1 tbsp. chopped pimientos

Combine cauliflower, water, salt, and dry mustard in a medium, microwaveable dish. Cover. Microwave on high 10 to 12 minutes. Stir occasionally. Remove cauliflower to a serving platter. Combine egg whites, parsley, and toasted oats and sprinkle over the cauliflower. Garnish with pimientos. Serves 4.

(Serving = 1 lean, fibrous vegetable)

Ratatouille

1 medium eggplant, peeled and cubed

2 medium zucchini, sliced

1 medium green pepper, thinly sliced

1 medium onion, sliced

1 clove garlic, minced

one 16-oz. can tomatoes

¼ cup chicken broth, defatted

½ tsp. basil

2 tbsp. chopped fresh parsley

Combine all ingredients, except parsley, in a heavy skillet. Cover and simmer over low heat for 15 minutes. Stir in parsley and cook 5 to 10 minutes or longer until vegetables are just tender. Serves 4. (Serving = 1 lean, fibrous vegetable)

Eggplant with Spaghetti Sauce

1 medium eggplant, peeled and sliced into ½ inch slices

1 stalk celery, chopped

1 carrot, shredded

1 cup chopped onion

¼ cup chicken broth, defatted

1 4-oz. can mushrooms, drained

¼ tbsp. garlic salt

1 tsp. Italian seasoning

¼ tsp. oregano leaves

1 8-oz. can tomatoes, drained and chopped

1 cup Spaghetti Sauce

Sprinkle the cut surfaces of the eggplant slices with salt. Let stand ½ hour. Rinse and drain slices. Place them in a 9" x 13" non-stick baking pan. Meanwhile, saute celery, carrot, and onion in broth in a medium skillet until tender. Add mushrooms, garlic salt, Italian seasoning, oregano, and tomatoes. Simmer 5 minutes. Spoon vegetable mixture on top of eggplant slices. Top with Spaghetti Sauce. Bake at 350 degrees 30 to 40 minutes until eggplant is tender. Serves 4. (Serving = 1 lean, fibrous vegetable)

Spaghetti Sauce

1 cup finely chopped onion
1 clove garlic, pressed
½ cup water
one 28-oz. can tomatoes, chopped
one 15-oz. can tomato sauce
¼ tsp. black pepper
1 tsp. oregano leaves
1 tsp. salt (optional)
1 tsp. basil
1 tsp. herb seasoning
1 tsp. celery flakes

In a large saucepan, saute onion and garlic in water until tender. Add remaining ingredients. Simmer uncovered until sauce has thickened (30 to 50 minutes). Makes 4 cups.

Green Beans Italiano

4 cups green beans, fresh or frozen
½ cup chopped onion
1 cup chopped tomatoes
⅓ cup water
½ tsp. Italian seasoning
½ tsp. oregano leaves
¼ tsp. seasoned salt

Combine all ingredients in a medium, microwaveable dish. Cover. Microwave on high until tender (14 to 16 minutes). Stir occasionally during heating. Serves 4.
(Serving = 1 lean, fibrous vegetable)

Fiesta Vegetables

3 medium green peppers, cut into strips
1 cup chopped onion
2 cups chopped tomatoes
½ cup water
½ tsp. cumin
1 tsp. oregano leaves
¼ tsp. seasoned salt
⅓ cup non-fat yogurt
1 tbsp. chopped fresh cilantro

Combine all ingredients, except yogurt, in a medium skillet. Saute vegetables until tender (6 to 8 minutes). Drain if necessary. Stir in non-fat yogurt and cilantro. Remove from heat and serve immediately. Serves 4.
(Serving = 1 lean, fibrous vegetable)

Vegetable Gumbo

2 cups okra, fresh or frozen

½ cup chopped onion

½ cup chopped green pepper

½ cup chicken broth, defatted

1 cup chopped tomatoes

½ tsp. marjoram

¼ tsp. garlic powder

½ tsp. seasoned salt

⅛ tsp. black pepper

If you are using fresh okra, cut the vegetable into ½-inch slices. Cook the okra in a small amount of boiling water for 10 minutes. Drain and rinse. For frozen okra, cook the vegetable according to package directions. Combine onion, green pepper, and broth. Saute until tender. Add okra, tomatoes, and remaining ingredients. Cook 3 to 5 minutes until heated. Serves 4.

(Serving = 1 lean, fibrous vegetable)

Spaghetti Squash

1 medium spaghetti squash

4 cups spaghetti sauce

Wash squash. Pierce and bake at 350 degrees for 1 to 1½ hours until soft. Remove squash from oven and cool slightly. Cut in half lengthwise and remove seeds and stringy membrane. Scoop out the pulp with a fork. The pulp resembles strands of spaghetti. Serve with spaghetti sauce. Serves 4.

(Serving = 2 lean, fibrous vegetables)

Spinach and Mushroom Saute

12 cups fresh spinach or 2 10-oz. packages frozen spinach
2 cups sliced fresh mushrooms
½ tsp. onion salt
¼ tsp. garlic powder
1 tsp. herb seasoning
⅛ tsp. crushed red pepper

Wash spinach thoroughly and drain. Combine all ingredients in a large skillet. Cover and simmer 10 to 15 minutes, stirring occasionally, until spinach is wilted and mushrooms are tender. Serves 4. (Serving = 1 lean, fibrous vegetable)

Spinach Pan Quiche

12 cups fresh spinach or 2 10-oz. packages frozen spinach
½ cup diced onion
¼ tsp. paprika
3 egg whites
½ tsp. garlic salt
4 tsp. lemon juice

Wash spinach thoroughly and drain. Put spinach, onion, and paprika in a large skillet. Cover and simmer 10 to 15 minutes until spinach is wilted. Increase heat and boil off excess liquid. Add egg whites, garlic salt, and lemon juice. Cook and stir until egg whites are scrambled. Serve immediately. Serves 4.

(Serving = 1 lean, fibrous vegetable)

Italian Stuffed Tomatoes

4 medium tomatoes

¼ cup chopped onion

1 cup shredded zucchini

2 cups sliced fresh mushrooms

¼ tsp. oregano leaves

1 tbsp. chopped fresh parsley

¼ tsp. garlic salt

1 egg white

1 tbsp. toasted oats

Cut tomatoes in half, crosswise. Scoop out soft pulp and drain liquid. Add tomato pulp, onion, zucchini, and mushrooms to a medium skillet. Cover and cook 6 to 8 minutes. Remove skillet from heat and drain off any excess liquid. Add oregano, fresh parsley, garlic salt, and egg white. Mix well and stuff tomato halves. Place stuffed tomatoes in a shallow, microwaveable dish. Sprinkle with toasted oats. Microwave uncovered for 5 to 6 minutes until tomatoes are soft. Serves 4. (Serving = 1 lean, fibrous vegetable)

Squash Medley

¼ cup sliced green onion

1 clove garlic, pressed

½ cup sliced celery

½ cup sliced carrots

½ cup julienned green pepper

½ cup chicken broth, defatted

3 cups sliced yellow squash

2 tbsp. low-salt soy sauce

¼ tsp. seasoned salt

½ tsp. basil

Saute green onion, garlic, celery, carrots, and green peppers in broth in a medium skillet until tender. Add squash, soy sauce, salt, and basil. Cook covered for 5 to 7 minutes until squash is tender. Serves 4. (Serving = 1 lean, fibrous vegetable)

Zucchini and Yellow Squash

2 cups sliced zucchini

2 cups sliced yellow squash

½ cup sliced onion

1 tbsp. lemon juice

3 tbsp. water

one 2-oz. jar pimientos, chopped

½ tsp. basil

½ tsp. seasoned salt

Combine all ingredients in a medium, microwaveable dish. Cover. Microwave on high until just tender (about 6 to 8 minutes). Stir occasionally during heating. Serves 4.
(Serving = 1 lean, fibrous vegetable)

Basil Vinaigrette

⅓ cup red wine vinegar

⅓ cup chicken broth

2 tbsp. basil

½ tsp. garlic salt

¼ tsp. black pepper

1 tsp. thyme leaves

Shake all ingredients in a small, covered jar. Refrigerate and use as needed. Makes ⅔ cup.

Herb Vinaigrette

⅔ cup cider vinegar

¼ cup water

2 tbsp. safflower oil

1 tsp. herb seasoning

1 tsp. garlic powder

½ tsp. paprika

1 tsp. Italian seasoning

Shake all ingredients in a small, covered jar. Refrigerate and use as needed. Makes 1 cup.

Appendix C

Recommended Products

Recommended Products

Skinfold calipers for measuring bodyfat and lean mass: An accurate tool for measuring bodyfat using skinfold calipers is the Parrillo Performance Bodystat Kit.

Vitamins: Parrillo Performance Essential Vitamin Formula™

Minerals: Parrillo Performance Mineral-Electrolyte Formula™

Lipotropics: Parrillo Performance Advanced Lipotropic Formula™

Endurance supplements (aspartates): Parrillo Performance Max Endurance Formula™

Carbohydrate supplements: Parrillo Performance ProCarb™

Protein supplements: Parrillo Performance Hi-Protein Powder,™ Vita-Herb Protein Powder, and Beverly International 100% Egg White Protein Powder

MCT oil: Parrillo Performance CapTri®

Evening primrose oil: Efamol

CoQ10: Twin Labs Coenzyme 10

Chromium: Twin Labs Chromium Picolinate

Desiccated Liver: Parrillo Performance Ultimate Amino
Beverly International Ultra 40

Garlic: Kyolic Aged Extract (Kyolic)

Please note: Cliff Sheats' Lean Bodies supplements and Parrillo Performance products may be
ordered by calling Lean Bodies at 1-800-697-LEAN. Other supplements can be found at most health
food stores or sports nutrition counters.

    Cliff Sheats' Lean Bodies products are formulated and produced with the assistance of Parrillo
Performance, Inc.

Appendix D

Food Composition Guide

Food Composition Guide

*Composition of Foods, 100 Grams, Edible Portion

FOOD	Calories	Protein	Fat	Carbohydrates	Sodium	Potassium	Calcium
Asparagus:							
Cooked spears, boiled, drained	20	2.2	0.2	3.6	1	183	21
Frozen-cuts and tips							
Cooked, boiled, drained	22	3.2	0.2	3.5	1	20	21
Frozen-spears							
Cooked, boiled, drained	23	3.2	0.2	3.8	1	238	
Barley, pearled, Light	349	8.2	1.0	78.8	3	160	160
Barley, pearled, Pot/Scotch	348	9.6	1.1	7.2		296	34
Bass:							
Black sea, raw	93	19.2	1.2		68	256	
Smallmouth, Largemouth, raw	104	18.9	2.6				
Striped, raw	105	8.9	2.7				
White, raw	98	18.0	2.3				
Beans, common, mature							
seeds, dry:							
White, raw	340	22.3	1.6	61.3	19	1196	144
White, cooked	118	7.8	0.6	21.2	7	416	50
Red, raw	343	22.5	1.5	61.9	10	984	110
Red, cooked	118	7.8	0.5	21.4	3	340	38
Pinto, calico, red Mexican, raw	349	22.9	1.2	63.7	10	984	135
Black, raw	339	22.3	1.5	61.2	25	1038	135
Beans, lima, mature							
seeds, dry:							
Raw	345	20.4	1.6	64.0	4	1529	72
Cooked	138	8.2	0.6	25.6	2	612	29

*Source: Composition of Foods, U.S. Department of Agriculture Handbook No. 8. *Agricultural Research Service. U.S. Department of Agriculture.*

Note: Conversions table located on page 281.

	Calories	Protein	Fat	Carbohydrates	Sodium	Potassium	Calcium
Beans, snap:							
Green, raw	32	1.9	0.2	7.1	7	243	56
Cooked, boiled, drained	25	1.6	0.2	5.4	4	151	50
Frozen, cut							
Cooked, boiled, drained	25	1.6	0.1	5.7	1	152	40
Frozen, French style							
Cooked, boiled, drained	26	1.6	0.1	6.0	2	136	38
Yellow or wax:							
Raw	27	1.7	0.2	6.0	7	243	56
Cooked, boiled, drained	22	1.4	0.2	4.6	3	151	50
Frozen, cut							
Cooked, boiled, drained	27	1.7	0.1	6.2	1	164	35
Beets, common, red:							
Raw	43	1.6	0.1	9.9	60	335	16
Cooked, boiled, drained	32	1.1	0.1	7.2	43	208	14
Beet greens, common:							
Raw	24	2.2	0.3	4.6	130	570	119
Cooked, boiled, drained	18	1.7	0.2	3.3	76	332	99
Bluefish, raw	117	20.5	3.3		74		23
Broadbeans, raw:							
Immature seeds	105	8.4	0.4	17.8	4	471	27
Mature seeds, dry	338	25.1	1.7	58.2			102
Broccoli:							
Raw spears	32	3.6	0.3	5.9	15	382	103
Cooked, boiled, drained	26	3.1	0.3	4.5	10	267	88
Frozen, chopped							
Cooked, boiled, drained	26	2.9	0.3	4.6	15	212	54

*Composition of Foods, 100 Grams, Edible Portion

	Calories	Protein	Fat	Carbohydrates	Sodium	Potassium	Calcium
Spears, cooked, boiled, drained	26	3.1	0.2	4.7	12	220	41
Brussels sprouts:							
Raw	45	4.9	0.4	8.3	14	390	36
Cooked, boiled, drained	36	4.2	0.4	6.4	10	273	32
Frozen, cooked, boiled, drained	33	3.2	0.2	6.5	14	295	21
Bulgur (parboiled wheat):							
Dry, commercial, made from-							
Club wheat	359	8.7	1.4	79.5		262	30
Hard red winter wheat	354	11.2	1.5	75.7		229	29
White wheat	357	10.3	1.2	78.1		310	36
Cabbage:							
Common varieties							
Raw	24	1.3	0.2	5.4	20	233	49
Cooked, boiled, drained							
Shredded	20	1.1	0.2	4.3	14	163	44
Wedges	18	1.0	0.2	4.0	13	151	42
Red, raw	31	2.0	0.2	6.9	26	268	42
Savoy, raw	24	2.4	0.2	4.6	22	269	67
Cabbage, Chinese (celery cabbage)							
Compact heading type, raw	14	1.2	0.1	3.0	23	253	43
Carrots							
Raw	42	1.1	0.2	9.7	47	341	37
Cooked, boiled, drained	31	0.9	0.2	7.1	33	222	33
Catfish, freshwater, raw	103	17.6	3.1		60	330	

*Source: Composition of Foods, U.S. Department of Agriculture Handbook No. 8. *Agricultural Research Service. U.S. Department of Agriculture.*

	Calories	*Protein*	*Fat*	*Carbohydrates*	*Sodium*	*Potassium*	*Calcium*
Cauliflower:							
Raw	27	2.7	0.2	5.2	13	295	25
Cooked, boiled, drained	22	2.3	0.2	4.1	9	206	21
Frozen, cooked, boiled, drained	18	1.9	0.2	3.3	10	207	17
Celery:							
Raw	17	0.9	0.1	3.9	126	341	39
Cooked, boiled, drained	14	0.8	0.1	3.1	88	239	31
Chicken:							
Light meat without skin, raw	117	23.4	1.9		50	320	11
Chickpeas, mature seeds,							
dry, raw	360	20.5	4.8	61	26	797	150
Cod, raw	78	17.6	0.3		70	382	10
Collards:							
Raw							
Leaves without stems	45	4.8	0.8	7.5		450	250
Including stems	40	3.6	0.7	7.2	43	401	203
Cooked, boiled, drained							
Leaves without stems, cooked							
in small amount of water	33	3.6	0.7	5.1		262	188
in large amount of water	31	3.4	0.7	4.8		243	177
Frozen, cooked, boiled, drained	30	2.9	0.4	5.6	16	236	176
Corn, sweet, white and							
yellow:							
Raw							
Cooked, boiled, drained	96	3.5	1.0	22.1	trace	280	3
Kernels, cut off cob	83	3.2	1.0	18.8	trace	165	3
Kernels, cooked on cob	91	3.3	1.0	21.0	trace	196	3

*Composition of Foods, 100 Grams, Edible Portion

	Calories	Protein	Fat	Carbohydrates	Sodium	Potassium	Calcium
Frozen							
Kernels, cut off cob	79	3.0	0.5	18.8	1	184	3
Kernels, cooked on cob	94	3.5	1.0	21.6	1	231	3
Corn grits, degermed and							
enriched:							
Dry form	362	8.7	0.8	78.1	1	80	4
Cooked	51	1.2	0.1	11.0	205	11	1
Cowpeas, including black-							
eyed peas:							
Immature seeds							
Frozen (black-eyed peas only)							
Cooked, boiled, drained	130	8.9	0.4	23.5	39	337	28
Mature seeds							
Raw	44	3.3	0.3	9.5	4	215	74
Cooked	34	2.6	0.3	7.0	3	196	17
Cucumbers:							
Not pared	15	0.9	0.1	3.4	6	160	25
Pared	14	0.6	0.1	3.2	6	160	17
Egg whites, fresh	51	10.9	trace	0.8	146	139	9
Eggplant:							
Raw	25	1.2	0.2	5.6	2	214	12
Cooked, boiled, drained	19	1.0	0.2	4.1	1	150	11
Endive (curly and							
escarole), raw	20	1.7	0.1	4.1	14	294	81
Flounder, cooked, baked	202	30.0	8.2		237	587	23

*Source: Composition of Foods, U.S. Department of Agriculture Handbook No. 8. *Agricultural Research Service. U.S. Department of Agriculture.*

	Calories	Protein	Fat	Carbohydrates	Sodium	Potassium	Calcium
Garbanzos, mature seeds,							
dry, raw	360	20.5	4.8	61	26	797	150
Grouper, incl. red, black							
and speckled							
Raw	87	19.3	0.5				
Haddock, raw	79	18.3	0.1		61	304	23
Halibut, Atlantic and							
Pacific , raw	100	20.9	1.2		54	449	13
Kale:							
Raw							
Leaves without stems, midribs	53	6.0	0.8	9.0	75	378	249
Cooked, boiled, drained							
Leaves without stems, midribs	39	4.5	0.7	6.1	43	221	187
Frozen							
Cooked, boiled, drained	31	3.0	0.5	5.4	21	193	121
Lake trout, raw	168	18.3	10.0				
Leeks, bulb and lower							
leaf portion							
Raw	52	2.2	0.3	11.2	5	347	52
Lentils, mature seeds, dry:							
Whole, raw	340	24.7	1.1	60.1	30	377	79
Whole, cooked	106	7.8	trace	19.3		249	25
Split, without seed coat, raw	345	24.7	0.9	61.8			46
Lettuce, raw:							
Butterhead, Boston, Bibb	14	1.2	0.2	2.5	9	264	35
Cos or Romaine	18	1.3	0.3	3.5	9	264	68
Looseleaf, or bunching varieties	18	1.3	0.3	3.5	9	264	68

*Composition of Foods, 100 Grams, Edible Portion

	Calories	Protein	Fat	Carbohydrates	Sodium	Potassium	Calcium
Mackerel, Atlantic, raw	191	19.0	12.2				5
Mackerel, Pacific, raw	159	21.9	7.3				8
Milk, cow:							
Fluid (pasteurized and raw)							
Skim	36	3.6	0.1	5.1	52	145	121
Dry							
Skim (non-fat solids), regular	363	35.9	0.8	52.3	532	1745	1308
Skim (non-fat solids), instant	359	35.8	0.7	51.6	526	1725	1293
Mushrooms, cultivated commercially:							
Raw	28	2.7	0.3	4.4	15	414	6
Canned, solids and liquid	17	1.9	0.1	2.4	400	197	6
Mustard greens:							
Raw	31	3.0	0.5	5.6	32	377	183
Cooked, boiled, drained	23	2.2	0.4	4.0	18	220	138
Frozen, cooked, boiled, drained	20	2.2	0.4	3.1	10	157	104
New Zealand spinach:							
Raw	19	2.2	0.3	3.1	159	795	58
Cooked, boiled, and drained	13	1.7	0.2	2.1	92	463	48
Oatmeal, or rolled oats:							
Dry form	390	14.2	7.4	68.2	2	352	53
Cooked	55	2.0	1.0	9.7	218	61	9
Ocean perch, raw	88	18.0	1.2		79	269	20
Onions, mature, dry:							
Raw	38	1.5	0.1	8.7	10	157	27

*Source: Composition of Foods, U.S. Department of Agriculture Handbook No. 8. *Agricultural Research Service. U.S. Department of Agriculture.*

	Calories	Protein	Fat	Carbohydrates	Sodium	Potassium	Calcium
Cooked, boiled, drained	29	1.2	0.1	6.5	7	110	24
Onions, young green							
(bunching varieties):							
Raw, bulb & entire top	36	1.5	0.2	8.2	5	231	51
Raw, bulb & white portion of top	45	1.1	0.2	10.5	5	231	40
Parsnips:							
Raw	76	1.7	0.5	17.5	12	541	50
Cooked, boiled, drained	66	1.5	0.5	14.9	8	379	45
Peas, edible-podded:							
Raw	53	3.4	0.2	12.0	170	62	
Cooked, boiled, drained	43	2.9	0.2	9.5	119	56	
Peas, green, immature:							
Raw	84	6.3	0.4	14.4	2	316	26
Cooked, boiled, drained	71	5.4	0.4	12.1	1	196	23
Frozen, cooked, boiled, drained	68	5.1	0.3	11.8	115	135	19
Peas and carrots, frozen:							
Cooked, boiled, drained	53	3.2	0.3	10.1	84	157	25
Peppers, sweet, garden							
varieties:							
Immature, green							
Raw	22	1.2	0.2	4.8	13	213	9
Cooked, boiled, drained	18	1.0	0.2	3.8	9	149	9
Perch:							
White, raw	118	19.3	4.0				
Yellow, raw	91	19.5	0.9		68	230	

*Composition of Foods, 100 Grams, Edible Portion

	Calories	Protein	Fat	Carbohydrates	Sodium	Potassium	Calcium
Pimientos, canned, solids and liquid	27	0.9	0.5	5.8			7
Pollock, raw	95	20.4	0.9		48	350	
Popcorn, popped, plain	386	12.7	5.0	76.7	3		11
Potatoes:							
Raw	76	2.1	0.1	17.1	3	407	7
Cooked							
Baked in skin	93	2.6	0.1	21.1	4	503	9
Boiled in skin	76	2.	0.1	17.1	3	407	7
Boiled, pared before cooking	65	1.9	0.1	14.5	2	285	6
Pumpkin:							
Raw	26	1.0	0.1	6.5	1	340	21
Canned	33	1.0	0.3	7.9	2	240	25
Radishes, raw							
Common	17	1.0	0.1	3.6	18	322	30
Oriental, diakon and Chinese	19	0.9	0.1	4.2		180	35
Red and gray snapper, raw	93	19.8	0.9		67	323	16
Rice:							
Brown, raw	360	7.5	1.9	77.4	9	214	32
Brown, cooked	119	2.5	0.6	25.5	282	70	12
Rutabagas:							
Raw	46	1.1	0.1	11.0	5	239	66
Cooked, boiled, drained	35	0.9	0.1	8.2	4	167	59
Salmon:							
Atlantic, raw	217	22.5	13.4		79		

*Source: Composition of Foods, U.S. Department of Agriculture Handbook No. 8. *Agricultural Research Service. U.S. Department of Agriculture.*

	Calories	Protein	Fat	Carbohydrates	Sodium	Potassium	Calcium
Pink (humpback), raw	119	20.0	3.7		64	306	
Sockeye (red),							
Canned, solids and liquid	171	20.3	9.3		522	344	
Seabass, white, raw	96	21.4	0.5				
Shad or American shad, raw	170	18.6	10.0		54	330	20
Shrimp:							
Raw	91	18.1	0.8	1.5	140	220	63
Canned							
Wet pack, solids and liquid	80	16.2	0.8	0.8	59		
Dry pack or drained solids of							
wet pack	116	24.2	1.1	0.7	122	115	
Soybeans, mature seeds,							
dry, raw	403	34.1	17.7	33.5	5	1677	226
Soybeans, mature seeds,							
dry, cooked	130	11.0	5.7	10.8	2	540	73
Spinach:							
Raw	26	3.2	0.3	4.3	71	470	93
Cooked, boiled, drained	23	3.0	0.3	3.6	50	324	93
Frozen, chopped							
Cooked, boiled, drained	23	3.0	0.3	3.7	52	333	113
Frozen, leaf							
Cooked, boiled, drained	24	2.9	0.3	3.9	49	362	105
Squash:							
Summer, all varieties							
Raw	19	1.1	0.1	4.2	1	202	28
Cooked, boiled, drained	14	0.9	0.1	3.1	1	141	25

*Composition of Foods, 100 Grams, Edible Portion

	Calories	Protein	Fat	Carbohydrates	Sodium	Potassium	Calcium
Crookneck and Straightneck, yellow, raw	20	1.2	0.2	4.3	1	202	28
Cooked, boiled, drained	15	1.0	0.2	3.1	1	141	25
Scallop varieties, white and pale green							
Raw	21	0.9	0.1	5.1	1	202	28
Cooked, boiled, drained	16	0.7	0.1	3.8	141	25	
Zucchini and Cocozelle, (Italian marrow type), green							
Raw	17	1.2	0.1	3.6	1	202	28
Cooked, boiled, drained	12	1.0	0.1	2.5	1	141	25
Winter, all varieties							
Raw	50	1.4	0.3	12.4	1	369	22
Cooked							
Baked	63	1.8	0.4	15.4	1	258	28
Boiled and mashed	38	1.1	0.3	9.2	1	258	20
Acorn							
Raw	44	1.5	0.1	11.2	1	384	31
Cooked							
Baked	55	1.9	0.1	14.0	1	480	28
Boiled and mashed	34	1.2	0.1	8.4	1	269	28
Butternut							
Raw	54	1.4	0.1	14.0	1	487	32
Cooked							
Baked	68	1.8	0.1	17.5	1	609	40

*Source: Composition of Foods, U.S. Department of Agriculture Handbook No. 8. *Agricultural Research Service. U.S. Department of Agriculture.*

	Calories	Protein	Fat	Carbohydrates	Sodium	Potassium	Calcium
Boiled and mashed	41	1.1	0.1	10.4	1	341	29
Hubbard							
Raw	39	1.4	0.3	9.4	1	217	19
Cooked							
Baked	50	1.8	0.4	11.7	1	271	24
Boiled and mashed	30	1.1	0.3	6.9	1	152	17
Squash, frozen							
Summer, Yellow Crookneck							
Cooked, boiled, drained	21	1.4	0.1	4.7	3	167	14
Winter							
Heated	38	1.2	0.3	9.2	1	207	25
Succotash (corn & lima beans)							
Frozen							
Cooked, boiled, drained	93	4.2	0.4	20.5	38	246	13
Sweet potatoes:							
Raw, all commercial varieties	114	1.7	0.4	26.3	10	243	32
Cooked, all commercial varieties							
Baked in skin	141	2.1	0.5	32.5	12	300	40
Boiled in skin	114	1.7	0.4	26.3	10	243	32
Swordfish, raw	118	19.2	4.0				19
Tomatoes, raw	22	1.1	0.2	4.7	3	244	13
Cooked, boiled	26	1.3	0.2	5.5	4	287	15
Canned, solids and liquid							
Regular pack	21	1.0	0.2	4.3	130	217	6
Dietary pack (low sodium)	20	1.0	0.2	4.2	3	217	6

*Composition of Foods, 100 Grams, Edible Portion

	Calories	Protein	Fat	Carbohydrates	Sodium	Potassium	Calcium
Tomato juice:							
Canned or bottled							
Regular pack	19	0.9	0.1	4.3	200	227	7
Dietary pack (low sodium)	19	0.8	0.1	4.3	3	227	7
Trout, brook, raw	101	19.2	2.1				
Trout, rainbow or steelhead, raw	195	21.5	11.4				
Tuna:							
Bluefin, raw	145	25.2	4.1				
Yellowfin, raw	133	24.7	3.0		37		
Canned in water, solids and liquid	127	28.0	0.8		41	279	16
Turkey, light meat, raw	116	24.6	1.2		51	320	
Turnips:							
Raw	30	1.0	0.2	6.6	49	268	39
Cooked, boiled, drained	23	0.8	0.2	4.9	34	188	35
Turnip greens, leaves including stems							
Raw	28	3.0	0.3	5.0			246
Cooked, boiled, drained, in small amount of water, short time	20	2.2	0.2	3.6			184
in large amount of water, long time	19	2.2	0.2	3.3			174
Canned, solids and liquids	18	1.5	0.3	3.2	236	243	100
Frozen, cooked, boiled, drained	23	2.5	0.3	3.9	17	149	118

*Source: Composition of Foods, U.S. Department of Agriculture Handbook No. 8. *Agricultural Research Service. U.S. Department of Agriculture.*

	Calories	Protein	Fat	Carbohydrates	Sodium	Potassium	Calcium
Vegetable juice cocktail, canned	17	0.9	0.1	3.6	200	221	12
Vegetables, mixed (carrots, corn, peas, green snap beans, lima beans) frozen Cooked, boiled, drained	64	3.2	0.3	13.4	53	191	25
Watercress, leaves with stems, raw	19	2.2	0.3	3.0	52	282	151
Wheat, shredded, without salt or other ingredients added	354	9.9	2.0	79.9	3	348	43
Whitefish, lake, raw	155	18.9	8.2		52	299	
Yam, tuber, raw	101	2.1	0.2	23.2		600	20
Yogurt, made from partially skimmed milk	50	3.4	1.7	5.2	51	143	120

Conversions

1 ounce = 28 grams

1 pound = 16 ounces = 453.59 grams

1 cup of water = 237 grams

1 fluid ounce of water = 30 grams

Appendix E

Participating Lean Bodies Restaurants

❧ *Participating Lean Bodies Restaurants*

Alabama

Athens

  Bonanza

Decatur

  Bonanza

Dothan

  Bonanza

Florence

  Bonanza

Huntsville

  Bonanza

Muscle Shoals

  Bonanza

Phenix City

  Bonanza

Talladega

  Bonanza

Arizona

Mesa

  Bonanza

Phoenix

  The Black-Eyed Pea

  Two Pesos

Scottsdale

  Two Pesos

Tempe

  Two Pesos

Arkansas

Batesville

  Bonanza

Bentonville

  Bonanza

Blytheville

  Bonanza

Camden

  Bonanza

Conway

  Bonanza

El Dorado

  Bonanza

Fayetteville

  Bonanza

Forrest City

  Bonanza

Ft. Smith

  Bonanza

Harrison

  Bonanza

Hot Springs
Bonanza

Jacksonville
Bonanza

Jonesboro
Bonanza

Little Rock
Black-Eyed Pea
Bonanza

Mountain Home
Bonanza

Paragould
Bonanza

Pocahontas
Bonanza

Rogers
Bonanza

Russellville
Bonanza

Searcy
Bonanza

Siloam Springs
Bonanza

Springdale
Bonanza

W. Memphis
Bonanza

California

Baldwin Park
Bonanza

Sacramento
The Black-Eyed Pea

Santa Clara
Bonanza

Colorado

Aurora
Bonanza

Denver
The Black-Eyed Pea

Lakewood
Bonanza

Thornton
Bonanza

Delaware

Dover
Bonanza

Milford
Bonanza

Millsboro
Bonanza

Newport
Bonanza

Florida

Miami
Bonanza

Orlando
The Black-Eyed Pea

Georgia

Atlanta
The Black-Eyed Pea
Two Pesos

Columbus
Bonanza

Duluth
The Black-Eyed Pea

Marietta
The Black-Eyed Pea

Norcross
The Black-Eyed Pea

Stone Mountain
The Black-Eyed Pea

Tucker
The Black-Eyed Pea

Idaho

Coeur d'Alene
Bonanza

Lewiston
Bonanza

Illinois

Anna
Bonanza

Benton
Bonanza

Bloomington
Bonanza

Carmi
Bonanza

Centralia
Bonanza

Champaign
Bonanza

Chicago
The Black-Eyed Pea
Bonanza

Decatur
Bonanza

East Moline
Bonanza

Effingham
Bonanza

Harrisburg
Bonanza

Highland
Bonanza

Lincoln
Bonanza

Marion
Bonanza

Mattoon
Bonanza

Mount Vernon
Bonanza

Springfield
Bonanza

Iowa

Ames
Bonanza

Cedar Falls
Bonanza

Cedar Rapids
Bonanza

Council Bluffs
Bonanza

Davenport
Bonanza

Des Moines
Bonanza

Dubuque
Bonanza

Ft. Dodge
Bonanza

Marshalltown
Bonanza

Mason City
Bonanza

Oskaloosa
Bonanza

Sioux City
Bonanza

Waterloo
Bonanza

Kansas

Dodge City
Bonanza

Emporia
Bonanza

Garden City
Bonanza

Hutchinson
Bonanza

Junction City
Bonanza

Kansas City
The Black-Eyed Pea

Lawrence
Bonanza

Manhattan
Bonanza

Pittsburg
Bonanza

Salina
Bonanza

Wichita
The Black-Eyed Pea
Bonanza

Kentucky

Florence
Bonanza
London
Bonanza
Madisonville
Bonanza
Newport
Bonanza
Somerset
Bonanza

Louisiana

Alexandria
Bonanza
Deridder
Bonanza
Houma
Bonanza
Lafayette
Bonanza
Lake Charles
Bonanza
Leesville
Bonanza
Monroe
Bonanza
Natchitoches
Bonanza

Opelousas
Bonanza
Ruston
Bonanza
Sulphur
Bonanza

Maine

Presque Isle
Bonanza
Rockland
Bonanza
Sanford
Bonanza

Maryland

Aberdeen
Bonanza
Baltimore
The Black-Eyed Pea
Elkton
Bonanza
Hagarstown
Bonanza
Pocomoke City
Bonanza
Salisbury
Bonanza

Washington DC
Bonanza

Michigan

Cadillac
Bonanza
Houghton
Bonanza
Marquette
Bonanza
Muskegon
Bonanza
Pittsfield
Bonanza
Traverse City
Bonanza
Warren
Bonanza

Minnesota

Apple Valley
Bonanza
Baxter
Bonanza
Bemidji
Bonanza
Burnsville
Bonanza

Coon Rapids
Bonanza

Detroit Lakes
Bonanza

Minneapolis
Two Pesos

New Ulk
Bonanza

Rochester
Bonanza

Spring Lake Park
Bonanza

St. Cloud
Two Pesos
Bonanza

Mississippi

Corinth
Bonanza

Hattiesburg
Bonanza

Jackson
Bonanza

Laurel
Bonanza

Meridian
Bonanza

Oxford
Bonanza

Pearl
Bonanza

Tupelo
Bonanza

Vicksburg
Bonanza

Missouri

Branson
Bonanza

Cape Girardeau
Bonanza

Independence
Bonanza

Joplin
Bonanza

Kansas City
The Black-Eyed Pea

Poplar Bluff
Bonanza

Sikeston
Bonanza

Springfield
Bonanza
Cheddars

St. Joseph
Bonanza

Nebraska

Beatrice
Bonanza

Bellevue
Bonanza

Columbus
Bonanza

Fremont
Bonanza

Grand Isle
Bonanza

Kearney
Bonanza

Lincoln
Bonanza

Norfolk
Bonanza

North Platte
Bonanza

Omaha
Bonanza

Scottsbluff
Bonanza

York
Bonanza

New Hampshire

Rochester
Bonanza

Laconia
Bonanza

New Jersey

Northfield

Bonanza

New Mexico

Albuquerque

The Black-Eyed Pea

Bonanza

New York

Plattsburg

Bonanza

North Dakota

Bismarck

Bonanza

Dickinson

Bonanza

Fargo

Bonanza

Grand Forks

Bonanza

Jamestown

Bonanza

Mandan

Bonanza

Nihot

Bonanza

Williston

Bonanza

Ohio

Barrie

Bonanza

Cambridge

Bonanza

Cincinnati

Bonanza

Fairfield

Bonanza

Kingston

Bonanza

Marietta

Bonanza

North Bay

Bonanza

North York

Bonanza

Sault Saint Marie

Bonanza

Springfield

Bonanza

St. Clairsville

Bonanza

Sudbury

Bonanza

Thunder Bay

Bonanza

Oklahoma

Oklahoma City

The Black -Eyed Pea

Tulsa

The Black-Eyed Pea

Pennsylvania

Berwick

Bonanza

Boyertown

Bonanza

Breezewood

Bonanza

Carlisle

Bonanza

Chambersburg

Bonanza

Dallas

Bonanza

Dubois

Bonanza

Ephraia

Bonanza

Frackville

Bonanza

Franklin

Bonanza

Gettysburg

Bonanza

Hanover

Bonanza

Heidelberg

Bonanza

Honaca

Bonanza

Lancaster

Bonanza

Lansdale

Bonanza

Lyndora

Bonanza

Mechanicsburg

Bonanza

New Columbia

Bonanza

Phoenixville

Bonanza

Pittson Township

Bonanza

Shahokin

Bonanza

Shippenville

Bonanza

Somerset

Bonanza

State College

Bonanza

Thorndale

Bonanza

Washington

Bonanza

Williamsport

Bonanza

South Dakota

Aberdeen

Bonanza

Brookings

Bonanza

Mitchell

Bonanza

Rapid City

Bonanza

Sioux Falls

Bonanza

Watertown

Bonanza

Yankton

Bonanza

Tennessee

Bartlett

The Black-Eyed Pea

Bristol

Bonanza

Dyersburg

Bonanza

Greeneville

Bonanza

Jackson

Bonanza

Kingsport

Bonanza

Martin

Bonanza

Memphis

The Black-Eyed Pea

Bonanza

Milan

Bonanza

Nashville

Bonanza

Paris

Bonanza

Savannah

Bonanza

Union City

Bonanza

Texas

Addison

The Black-Eyed Pea

Addison

Chili's Grill & Bar

Amarillo

The Black-Eyed Pea

Arlington
  Chili's Grill & Bar
  The Black-Eyed Pea
  Two Pesos
  Pulido's
  Cheddars
Austin
  The Black-Eyed Pea
Beaumont
  The Black-Eyed Pea
  Bonanza
Bedford
  Chili's Grill & Bar
Brownsville
  Bonanza
Brownwood
  Pulido's
Bryan College Station
  The Black-Eyed Pea
  Two Pesos
Carrollton
  Chili's Grill & Bar
  The Black-Eyed Pea
Cleburne
  Pulido's
Conroe
  The Black-Eyed Pea
Corpus Christi
  The Black-Eyed Pea
Dallas
  The Black-Eyed Pea

Bonanza
  Cheddars
  Ming Garden
  Two Pesos
  Zucchini's
Denton
  The Black-Eyed Pea
Eastland
  Pulido's
Fort Worth
  The Black-Eyed Pea
  Two Pesos
  Pulido's
  Cheddars
Galveston
  Two Pesos
Garland
  The Black-Eyed Pea
  Bonanza
Greenville
  Chili's Grill & Bar
  Bonanza
Harlingen
  Bonanza
Houston
  The Black-Eyed Pea
  Two Pesos
Humble
  The Black-Eyed Pea
Hurst
  The Black-Eyed Pea

Pulido's
Irving
  The Black-Eyed Pea
  Two Pesos
  Pulido's
Killeen
  Bonanza
Kingsville
  Bonanza
Lewisville
  The Black-Eyed Pea
  Bonanza
Longview
  Bonanza
Lubbock
  The Black-Eyed Pea
McAllen
  Bonanza
Mesquite
  The Black-Eyed Pea
Mineral Wells
  Pulido's
Missouri City
  The Black-Eyed Pea
North Richland Hills
  Two Pesos
  Pulido's
Pasadena
  The Black-Eyed Pea
Plano
  The Black-Eyed Pea

Richardson

   Chili's Grill & Bar

San Antonio

   The Black-Eyed Pea

   Bonanza

Stephenville

   Pulido's

Texarkana

   Bonanza

Tyler

   The Black-Eyed Pea

Weatherford

   Pulido's

Webster

   The Black-Eyed Pea

   Two Pesos

Weslaco

   Bonanza

Wichita Falls

   Bonanza

Vermont

Burlington

   Bonanza

Virginia

Abingdon

   Bonanza

Cedar Bluff

   Bonanza

Charlottesville

   Bonanza

Lebanon

   Bonanza

Newport News

   Cheddars

Radford

   Bonanza

Staunton

   Bonanza

Waynesboro

   Bonanza

Winchester

   Bonanza

Wise

   Bonanza

Washington

Kennewick

   Bonanza

Spokane

   Bonanza

Washington D. C.

   The Black-Eyed Pea

West Virginia

Barboursville

   Bananza

Bridgeport

   Bonanza

Charleston

   Bonanza

Fairmont

   Bonanza

Horgantown

   Bonanza

Huntington

   Bonanza

Lewisburg

   Bonanza

Lybrurn

   Bonanza

Madison

   Bonanza

Morgantown

   Bonanza

Parkersburg

   Bonanza

St. Albans

   Bonanza

Vienna

   Bonanza

Welch

   Bonanza

Weston Place

   Bonanza

Wisconsin

Appleton

Bonanza

Eau Claire

Bonanza

Fond Du Lac

Bonanza

Green Bay

Bonanza

Janesville

Bonanza

Onalaska

Bonanza

Oshkosh

Bonanza

Wausau

Bonanza

Wyoming

Cody

Bonanza

For updates on participating Lean Bodies restaurants, call (800) 875-3346.

Glossary

Absorption. The process by which nutrients pass through the intestines and enter the bloodstream for use by the body.

Amino acids. Building blocks of protein necessary for growth and metabolism.

Anabolism. The building of muscle tissue.

Antibodies. Proteins found in the blood which combat disease.

Antioxidant. A special class of nutrients that fight "free radicals," a group of cells that damage otherwise healthy cells.

Atherosclerosis. Hardening of the arteries caused by cholesterol and fats deposited in the arteries and oxidized there.

Bioavailability. How well vitamins and minerals are absorbed from the foods we eat.

Biochemical individuality. Physiological differences that exist in every human being.

Body composition. The ratio of lean mass (muscle) to bodyfat.

Bodyfat. Stored fat which is usually deposited around the hips, thighs, and abdomen.

Calorie. A measure of a unit of energy.

Carbohydrates. Food group that serves as an energy source for the body.

Carcinogens. Agents that cause cancer.

Catabolism. The breaking down of muscle tissue in response to exercise.

Cholesterol. A fatty substance found in some foods and manufactured by the body for many vital functions.

Cross-linking. A reaction in cell membranes thought to be responsible for hardening of the arteries, skin wrinkling, and cataracts.

Cruciferous vegetables. Vegetables that contain indoles, compounds that seem to protect against cancer. Broccoli, cauliflower, cabbage, and watercress are cruciferous vegetables.

Deficiency. Condition in which a nutrient or a group of nutrients is lacking.

Digestion. The breakdown of foods by enzymes so that nutrients can be absorbed by the body.

Dispensable amino acids. Amino acids that the body can synthesize on its own.

Disaccharide. A type of simple sugar constructed of double molecules of glucose.

Diuretics. Drugs that increase the rate of urine formation in the body.

Electrolytes. Minerals that are responsible for maintaining the fluid balance inside and outside cells.

Enzyme. A protein that brings about chemical changes without being affected itself.

Essential fatty acids (EFAs). Vitamin-like substances that have a protective effect on the body. They are called essential because the body cannot manufacture them. They must be obtained from food.

Famine/fat acceleration. A physiological defense mechanism involving the buildup of fat by the body following a period of caloric restriction.

Fatty acids. Components of either dietary fat or bodyfat.

Free radicals. Cellular aberrations, formed when molecules somehow come up with an odd number of electrons. These cells destroy healthy cells by robbing them of oxygen, and this robbery weakens the immune system. Normally, free radicals are not a problem because they are captured by the body's own army of antioxidants. Trouble arises, however, when free radicals outnumber antioxidants – a situation that results from aging and exposure to pollutants and toxins. Unchecked, free radicals roam the body, scavenging for oxygen and ultimately creating the type of cell damage associated with arthritis, cancer, heart disease, and other degenerative diseases.

Fructose. A monosaccharide found in fruit and fruit juices.

Galactose. A monosaccharide that is a part of lactose.

Glucagon. A hormone responsible for unlocking fat stores.

Glucose. Blood sugar.

Glucose tolerance. The ability to transport blood glucose into cells for use by the body.

Glycogen. Stored carbohydrate in the muscles and liver.

HDL (high density lipoprotein). A type of cholesterol in the blood that has a protective effect against the buildup of plaque in the arteries.

Heme iron. Iron found in animal protein.

Hemoglobin. A protein in red blood cells that transports oxygen from the lungs to the rest of the body.

Hormones. Chemicals that are secreted in body fluids and carried to organs to produce specific metabolic effects.

Hydrostatic underwater weighing. An accurate test for measuring bodyfat that immerses the subject underwater and calculates body composition by using a certain formula.

Hypoglycemia. Low blood sugar.

Immune system. A complex network of various types of cells and organs that work together to fight disease, from the common cold to deadly cancers. Proper nutrition is the most powerful way to keep your immune system strong. And a strong immune system is your fortress against disease.

Indispensable amino acids. Amino acids derived from animal sources of protein.

Indole. Compounds in cruciferous vegetables that have cancer-protective effects.

Insulin. A hormone involved in glucose metabolism, protein synthesis, and fat formation.

Lactose. The simple sugar found in milk.

Lean, fibrous vegetables. A type of complex carbohydrate that is high in fiber and minerals and low in calories.

Lean mass. The amount of muscle on your body.

LCT (long chain triglyceride). Another name for bodyfat and conventional dietary fat such as salad oil and margarine.

Leukocytes. A type of white blood cell that plays a major role in warding off infection. Leukocytes destroy bacteria and eat cellular debris at inflamed areas, among other functions.

Lipoprotein lipase (LPL). An enzyme governing fat storage. Repetitive low-calorie dieting causes the body to produce more LPL, and more bodyfat is produced and stored as a result.

Lipotropic. A fat-burning agent.

Low density lipoproteins (LDL). A type of cholesterol in the blood. High levels contribute to coronary heart disease.

Lymphocytes. A type of white blood cell formed in the lymphatic system. About 20 percent to 30 percent of the white blood cells in the body are lymphocytes.

Macrophages. Cells involved in the production of antibodies.

MCT oil (medium chain triglyceride oil). A dietary fat metabolized in such a way that very little is stored as bodyfat.

Maltose. A disaccharide found in plants during the early stages of germination.

Metabolic rate. The speed at which your body burns calories.

Metabolic roll. Condition in which the metabolism runs efficiently enough to burn fat.

Metabolism. The physiological process that converts food to energy so that your body can function.

Metabolic optimizers. A class of supplemental nutrients that enhance athletic performance.

Mineral. Inorganic nutrients needed by the body for a wide range of enzymatic and metabolic functions.

Mitochondria. The part of the cell where nutrients are converted to energy.

Mock meal. A beverage consisting of a carbohydrate and protein supplement used on the Lean Bodies program in midmorning and midafternoon to sustain energy levels.

Monosaccharide. A type of simple sugar constructed of a single molecule of glucose.

Monounsaturated fat. Fatty acids that lack two hydrogen atoms. Found in such foods as olive oil, olives, avocados, cashew nuts, and cold-water fish such as salmon, mackerel, halibut, and swordfish.

Neurotransmitters. Chemicals that relay nerve impulses.

Nitrogen balance. A measurement of whether you are losing or gaining lean muscle mass.

Nonheme iron. Type of iron found in plants.

Nutrition. The use of food for growth and development.

Omega-3 fatty acids. Essential fats found in fish that appear to prevent blood clots and the build-up of plaque on arterial walls. Omega-3 fatty acids also play a role in strengthening the immune system.

Oxidation. A chemical process in which oxygen combines with another substance, which is changed to another form.

Planned cheat. Planning to eat a treat on a certain day, at a certain time – without eating on impulse.

Polysaccharide. Multiple number of sugar molecules linked together in a long chain. Complex carbohydrates are polysaccharides.

Polyunsaturated fat. A fatty acid that lacks four or more hydrogen atoms. Found in fish and in most vegetable oils.

Prostaglandins. Hormone-like substances that regulate nearly every system in the body.

Protein. Food group necessary for growth and repair of body tissues.

Protein quality. A rating based on the number of indispensable amino acids present, digestibility, and absorbability.

Recommended dietary allowances (RDA). The amount of nutrients that should be taken by healthy individuals to prevent disease.

Saturated fat. A fatty acid that carries the maximum number of hydrogen atoms. Saturated fats are solid at room temperature.

Simple sugars. A type of carbohydrate that is constructed of either single or double molecules of glucose.

Skinfold calipers. The measurement of skinfold thicknesses using a special tool.

Specific dynamic action. The ability of certain foods to increase the metabolic rate after a meal is consumed.

Starchy carbohydrates. A natural complex carbohydrate.

T-cells. White blood cells that kill invading agents.

Thermogenesis. The production of body heat – a process that increases oxygen consumption and boosts the metabolic rate.

Trace mineral. An element present in small quantities in food yet that is vital to health.

Triglycerides. Fats that circulate in the blood until they are deposited in fat cells.

Ultrasound. A method of measuring body composition.

Unsaturated fat. Fats that are liquid at room temperature. Unsaturated fats are a source of essential fatty acids.

Vitamins. Organic substances found in food that perform many vital functions in the body.

Water-insoluble fiber. A type of fiber that supplies bulk to keep foods moving through the digestive system.

Water-soluble fiber. A type of fiber in grains, legumes, and carrots that has been shown to reduce cholesterol and slow the release of glucose into the bloodstream.

Index

A

Absorption, 112, 296

Adolescents, on Lean Bodies program, 206-7

Aerobic dancing, 144, 152-53

Aerobic exercise, 23-25, 141.
  See also Exercise; Exercise plan
  and aging, 194-95
  for arthritic patients, 144
  benefits of, 24, 141-42
  pre-breakfast, 103
  combining with weight
     training, 143-44
  duration and timing of, 24-25
  step aerobics, 152-53
  target heart rate in, 142
  types of, 24, 141, 144

Aging
  and aerobics, 194-95
  and bone mineral loss, 150
  healthy, 192-95
  and osteoporosis, 111, 125, 126,
     129, 132, 150, 172
  and weight training, 194-95

Alanine, 35

Alcohol, 210

Amino acids, 29, 296
  branched-chain, 180
  dispensable, 34, 35-36, 297

indispensable, 34-35, 300

Amphetamines, 17

Anabolism, 31, 296

Anemia, 39

iron deficiency, 127

megoblastic, 117-118

pernicious, 118

Antibodies, 33, 296

Antioxidants, 36, 193-94, 214, 296, 298

Arachidonic acid, 58

Arginine, 34, 181

Argine pyroglutamate, 181

Arthritis, and exercise, 144

Asparagus

Asparagus Oriental, 251-52

Asparagus Salad Vinaigrette, 245-46

Aspartates, 179

athletic need for, 179

supplements, 179

Aspartic acid, 35

Atherosclerosis, 116, 119, 296

Athletic needs

carbohydrates, 176

and gaining lean mass, 172-74

and meeting training needs, 181-82

metabolic optimizers, 178-81

nutritional needs of, 170-82

performance nutrients, 174-76

proteins, 172

vitamins and minerals, 177-78

B

Baked Potatoes with Tangy Toppers, 243

Bananas, 208

Barbecued Shrimp, 222

Basal Metabolic Rate (BMR), 190

Basil Vinaigrette, 261-62

B-complex vitamins, 114-18, 178. *See also* Cobalamin; Niacin; Pyroxidine; Riboflavin; Thiamine

athletic need for, 178

deficiency of, 177

sources of, 177

Beans

Beans and Rice Creole, 244-45

Hickory-Smoked Pinto Beans, 241-42

Navy Bean Soup and Vegetables, 236-37

Southern Salad, 233

Turkey and Vegetable Bisque, 232-33

Turkey Chili, 226

Beef, 39

Beets l'Orange, 252

Beri beri, 53

Beta carotene

anti-cancer effects of, 114, 192

as antioxidant, 193, 214

functions of, 114

Betaine, 134

Bicycling, 141, 153

stationary, 144, 153, 215

recumbent, 215

Bioavailability, 112, 296

Biochemical individuality, 112, 296

Biochemistry, changing your, 19-25

Biotin, 133

Blood ammonia, 179

Blood sugar. *See* Glucose

Body composition, 296

    methods for determining, 70-71

Bodyfat, 296-97

    accelerating loss, 102-6

    desirable percentages of, 7

    distribution of, 214

    eating to lose, 1-2

    using MCT oil to burn, 66

Bone mass. *See also* Osteoporosis

    and calcium supplementation, 125

    and exercise, 125-26

Boron

    food sources of, 129

    function of, 129

    supplementation, 129

Branched-chain amino acids, 180

Breakfast, 207, 208

    aerobic exercise before, 103

Broccoli

    Broccoli Italiano, 253

    Spicy Vegetables, 252-53

Brown rice. *See* Rice

Brown Rice and Mushrooms, 239

Brown Rice Supreme, 238-39

Bucci, Luke, 135

Bulking agents, 17-18

Business travel, exercise program on,
    216

C

Cabbage, 110

    Caraway Cabbage, 253

Caesar Salad, 248-49

Caffeine, 39

Cajun-Style Fish, 221

Calcium

    bioavailability of, 125

    deficiencies of, 111, 126

    food sources of, 37, 125

    functions of, 124-25

    loss of, and protein and phosphorus,
        172

    need for magnesium for metabolism
        of, 126

    supplementation, 125

Calories, 297

    and aerobic exercise, 23-24

    gradually increasing your, 19-21

    daily needs for optimum fueling,
        189-190

    spreading throughout day, 21-22

Cancer, 192

    and beta-carotene, 114, 192

    colon, 46-48, 53

    and exercise, 145

    and nutritional supplements, 111

    and Vitamin A, 114

Canola oil, 62, 212

CapTri, 62, 264

Caraway Cabbage, 253

Carbohydrates, 44-45, 297

    athletic need for, 176

    complex, 45, 48

conversion factor, 46-48

excluding from meal plan, 74-75, 105

fiber link, 52-54

impact of, on metabolism, 32

in lean, fibrous vegetables, 51-52

processed, 50

starchy, 48, 49-50, 74-75, 90, 304

simple sugars 45-46, 304

supplements, 264

Carcinogens, 297

Cardiovascular disease, 30

in diabetes, 147

and exercise, 146

risk factors for, 15

saturated fats in, 30

Carnitine shuttle, 65

Carrots

Carrots with Ginger, 254

Spicy Vegetables, 252-53

Catabolism, 31, 297

Catabolism/anabolism cycle, importance of protein in, 31-32

Cauliflower with Toasted Oats, 254

Cellular health, 59

Cellular immunity, 33-34

Cellular level fats, 64-65

Cellulose, 54

Chicken. *See also* Turkey

Chicken and Rice Soup, 230-31

Chicken Broth, 230

Potato Soup with Chicken, 231-32

Savory Poultry Strips, 227-28

Smothered Chicken, 225-26

as source of protein, 36, 37

Chile

Turkey Chili, 226

Chloride, 178

athletic need for, 178

deficiency of, 178

Cholesterol, 30, 136, 297

and CoQ10, 134-35

desired level, 12n

and exercise, 145-46

HDL, 136, 141, 146, 212, 299

LDL, 21, 118-19, 136, 146, 208, 301

and Vitamin C, 118-19

Choline, 133-34

synthesis of, 35

Chromium, 178, 265

function of, 130-31, 178

supplementation, 130, 131, 178

Chromium picolinate, 178

Chronic fatigue syndrome (CFS), 75

Cobalamin (Vitamin B-12), 38, 117-18

deficiencies, 117, 118

food sources, 38, 39, 117, 118

functions of, 117-18

Coenzyme Q10 (CoQ10), 134-35, 264

Coffee, 39-40

Collagen, 31, 36, 118

Colon cancer, risk of, 37-39, 54

Complex carbohydrates, 45, 48-49

Condiments, shopping for, 91

Conversion factor, 46-48

Cooking

in bulk, 91-92

and destruction of nutrients, 112,
117, 127
CoQ10, 134-35, 264
Corn
Festive Corn, 240
Tomato and Corn Soup, 238
Coronary heart disease. *See* Cardiovas
cular disease
Coronary thrombosis, 29
Cross country ski machines, 144, 154
Cross-linking, 194, 297
Cruciferous vegetables, 51, 297
Cysteine, 35
Cystine, 35

dangers in, 17-19
problems with, 13-16
Diet pills, dangers from, 9-10
Diet soft drinks, 209
Digestion, 297
Digestive juices, and low-calorie diets,
15
Disaccharides, 45-46, 298
Dispensable amino acids, 34, 35-36,
297
Distilled water, 40, 211
Diuretics, 18, 127, 298
DNA, 29

D

Dairy products, 125
on the Lean Bodies program, 48
sources of, 91
Deficiency, 297
Dehydration, 39
Depression, 148-49
Desiccated liver, 180-81, 265
Diabetes, 30
and chromium supplementation,
130, 131
and exercise, 147-48
and fiber, 194
and Lean Body program, 11-12
Dietary deficiencies, 110-11
Diet drugs, 17
Dieting

E

Eat, permission to, 3-5
Eating
to lose bodyfat, 1-2
in restaurants, 93-95, 208-209
Edema, 33
EFAs. *See* Essential fatty acids (EFAs)
Eggplant
Eggplant with Spaghetti Sauce,
255-56
Ratatouille, 255
Eggs
Egg White Casserole, 219
Egg White Scramble, 218
Potato Deviled Eggs, 218
Spinach Pan Quiche, 259
as source of protein, 36
Egg whites

commercially frozen, 207-8

as source of protein, 37

Electrolytes, 124, 178, 298

athletic need for, 178

deficiency of, 178

Emotional health, and exercise, 148-49

Emulsification, 63

Endocrine system disorders, 190-91

Endorphins, 35

Endurance supplements, 264

Energy, food combining for constant,
71-72

Enriched, 211-12

Enzyme, 298

Ershoff, B. H., 180-81

Essential fat, 7

Essential fatty acids (EFAs), 58, 59-60,
212, 298

and blood pressure, 193

deficiencies in, 60-61

and timing, 212

Estrogen, 129

Evening Primrose oil, 60, 61, 62, 264

Exercise, 140-144. See also Aerobic
exercise; Athletic needs; Weight
training

and bone mass, 125-26

determining goals in, 151

and emotional health, 148-49

excessive, 18-19

health benefits of, 144-51

on Lean Bodies program, 215

and metabolism, 23-24

and nutrient need, 112

scheduling, 215

secrets of success, 164-66

side effects of, 120-21

Exercise plan

and business travel, 216

adding weight training to, 158-60

designing your, 151-58

sticking to, 163-64

Exercise videos, 153

F

Famine/fat acceleration cycle, 14, 298

Fancy Tuna Salad, 224-25

Fast foods, 208-9

Fasting, 17

Fat(s), 6. See also Fatty acids

at cellular level, 64-65

chemical composition of, 58-60

essential, 7

MCT oil as, 62-64, 66

monounsaturated, 59, 302

polysaturated, 59, 303

proper amount of, 61-62

saturated, 30, 39, 59, 212, 304

sources of, 91

stored, 6-7

subcutaneous, 6

unsaturated, 59-60, 304

Fat burning, maximizing, 24-25

Fatigue, 10-11

Fat mobilization, 59

Fatty acids, 37-38, 58-59, 298 (cont).

Fatty acids (*cont*)

See also Essential fatty acids; Fats

monounsaturated, 59, 303

omega-3, 37, 58, 210, 303

polyunsaturated, 59, 303

Festive Corn, 240

Fiber, 52-55

sources of, 54

water-insoluble, 54, 305

water-soluble, 54, 305

Fiesta Vegetables, 257

Fish. *See also* Shrimp

Cajun-Style Fish, 221

Fancy Tuna Salad, 224-25

on Lean Bodies program, 38

Mexican Fish Fillets, 219-20

Seasoned Fish Fillets with Spinach, 220-21

as source of protein, 36, 37

Tuna Oriental, 223

Flaxseed oil, 60, 62

Folic acid, 111

Food composition guide, 264-81

Foods

choosing metabolic-activating, 22-23

grading protein quality of, 36

Framingham Heart Study, 15

Free radicals, 298-99

Freezing, tips for, 92-93

Fructose, 45, 47, 299

Fruits

on the Lean Bodies program, 48

and promotion of body fat, 46-47

G

Gala Cole Slaw, 246-47

Galactose, 45, 46, 299

Gallbladder disease, 15

Gamma-linolenic acid, 60

Garlic, 135-36, 265

as antioxidant, 214

function of, 135-36

supplementation, 136

Glucagon, 46, 66, 103, 299

Glucose, 44, 45, 46, 147, 176, 299

Glucose tolerance, 194, 299

and chromium supplementation, 130

Glutamic acid, 35

Glycine, 35, 131

Glycogen, 176, 299

Green Beans

Green Beans Italiano, 257

Potato and Green Bean Salad, 234

Guar gum, 17

Gums, 54

H

Hain All-Blend, 62

HDL. *See* High density lipoproteins (HDLs)

Heart disease. *See* Cardiovascular disease

Heme iron, 299

Hemicelluloses, 54

Hemoglobin, 127, 299

Herbed Potato Skins, 242-43

Herb Vinaigrette, 262

Hickory-Smoked Pinto Beans, 241-42

High blood pressure. *See* Hypertension

High-density lipoproteins (HDLs),
  136, 141, 146, 299
  desirable ranges for, 212

Histidine, 35

Homocysteine, 116-17

Hormones, 299

Human growth hormone (HGH), 181

Hydralazine, 117

Hydrophilic, 33

Hydrostatic underwater weighing, 70,
  299-300

Hydroxyproline, 36

Hypertension, 30, 193
  and exercise, 149

Hypoglycemia, 170, 213-14, 300

I

Ideal projected bodyweight (BW), 190

Immune system, 193, 300
  and aging, 192
  and beta carotene, 114
  and iron, 128
  and nutrition, 214
  and proteins, 33-34
  and Vitamin A, 114

Impulsive eating, 189

Indispensable amino acids, 34, 35, 300

Indole, 300

Inositol, 134

Insulin, 46, 103, 132, 171-72, 180,
  300

Interleukin, 120

Intrinsic factor, 118

Iron, 177-78
  athletic need for, 178-79
  deficiency of, 111, 127-28, 177
  function of, 127, 128
  heme, 299
  improving absorption of, 129
  nonheme, 302
  sources of, 38, 129, 177

Isoleucine, 35, 180

Italian Salad, 248

Italian Stuffed Tomatoes, 260

J

Jalapeno Tomato Sauce, 220

Jogging, 141, 154-55

K

Ketones, 65

Ketosis, 66

Kyolic aged garlic extract, 136

L

Lactate, 128

Lacto-ovo-vegetarians, 213

Lactose, 46, 300

  intolerance of, 46

Lamb, 208

Lau, B., 136

Laxatives, 127, 211

  abuse of, 18

L-carnitine, 36, 134

LCT. *See* Long chain triglyceride
  (LCTs)

LDL. *See* Low density lipoproteins
  (LDLs)

Lean, fibrous vegetables, 48-49, 51-52,
  300

  sources of, 90-91

Lean Bodies Cookbook, 5

Lean Bodies program

  amount of fat in, 61-62

  basis for, 3, 16

  breakfast on, 207, 208

  carbohydrates in, 49-50

  choosing metabolic-activating foods
    in, 22-23

  daily menu, 73

  dairy products on, 48

  and eating out, 93-95, 208-9

  exercise in, 23-25, 140-66

  expectations from, 8

  fish on, 38

  focus on losing bodyfat in, 6-8

  food classification in, 22-23

  food preparation in, 92-93

  fruits on, 48

  increasing calories in, 19-21

lean cooking in bulk, 91-92

lean, fibrous vegetables in, 48, 51-
  52, 90-91

lifestyle change in, 186-95

meal planning, 74-89, 104-5,
  173-74

mock meals in, 72,74

need for support, 95-97

nutritional stress in, 5

principles in, 19-25

Program I, 74-89, 102

Program II, 102-5

Program III, 105-7

proteins in, 36-38, 90

questions on, 206-16

recipes for, 218-62

shopping list for, 90-91

spreading out daily calories on,
  21- 22

weight gain on, 206

Lean cooking, in bulk, 91-92

Lean mass, 7, 300

  gaining, 10, 170-73

  menu plan for gaining, 173-74

Lean proteins, sources of, 90

Lean Thousand Island Dressing, 224

Lemon, Peter W. R., 171

Lemon Mustard Vinaigrette, 249-50

Leucine, 35, 180

Leukocytes, 34, 300-301

Lignins, 54

Linoleic acid, 58, 60, 193

Linolenic acid, 58

Linseed oil, 62

Lipid peroxides, 193-94

Lipoprotein lipase (LPL), 15, 301

Lipotropics, 133-34, 264, 301

   deficiency of, 133-34

   function of, 133

   supplements, 210

Liquid diets, problems with, 9, 16

Long chain triglycerides (LCTs), 300

   digestion of, 63-65

Low blood sugar, correcting, 213-14

Low-calorie diets

   impact on metabolism, 14

   problems with, 5-6, 111

   side effects of, 15-16

Low-density lipoproteins (LDLs), 21, 119, 136, 146, 208, 301

Low protein diets, adverse effects of, 30-34

Lymphocytes, 33, 301

Lysine, 34, 36, 181

M

Macrobiotic diet, 96-97

Macrophages, 33-34, 289

Magnesium, 36, 178

   athletic need for, 178

   deficiency of, 40, 111, 126, 178

   food sources of, 126

   function of, 126

Maltodextrin, 72

Maltose, 46, 301

Manganese

   deficiency of, 132

   function of, 131-32

Marinated Vegetable Salad, 247

Mashed Potatoes, 243-44

Mayo, Charles, 53

MCT oil, 62-64, 103, 105, 264, 301

   athletic use of, 181

   calories in, 212

   and fat gain, 212-13

   in place of other fats, 213

   using to burn bodyfat, 66

Meal plans

   adding foods back in, 187-88

   dropping carbohydrates from, 74-75, 105

   for lean mass gain, 173-74

   for Program 1, 74-89

   for Program II, 104-5

   for Program III, 106

Men

   meal plans for, 83-89

   minimum pace required to achieve target heart rate, 157-58

Meniere's Syndrome, 190

Mental attitude, and exercise success, 165-66

Metabolic activating foods, 22-23

Metabolic activator, 33

Metabolic optimizers, 178-81, 302

Metabolic rate, 301

Metabolic roll, 22, 301

Metabolism, 301-3

   and aging, 206

   and exercise, 23-24

impact of low-calorie diets on, 14

impact of protein on, 32

and MCT oil, 64

signs of faster, 20-21

Methionine, 34, 36

Methylcellulose, 17

Mexican Fish Fillets, 219-20

Milks. *See also* Dairy products

soy, 208-9

Minerals, 124, 264, 302

boron, 129

calcium, 38, 124-26, 172

chloride, 178

chromium, 130-31, 178, 265

coenzyme Q10 (CoQ10), 134-35, 264

garlic, 135-36, 214, 265

iron, 39, 127-29, 178-79, 299, 302

lipotropics, 133-34, 210, 264, 289

magnesium, 36, 40, 126, 178

manganese, 131-32

potassium, 74, 126-27, 178, 208, 211

selenium, 38, 132, 214

sodium, 127, 178, 210-11

trace, 304

zinc, 38, 132-33, 178

Mini meals, 72. *See also* Mock meals

Minted Peas, 241

Mitochrondria, 65, 302

Mock meals, 72, 302

number of daily, 208

preparing, 72,74

Monosaccharide, 45, 302

Monosaccharide glucose, 45

Monounsaturated fat, 302

Mucilages, 54

Muscle, and burning body fat, 172

Muscular definition, 214

Mushrooms

Brown Rice and Mushrooms, 239

Spinach and Mushroom Saute, 259

Myelin, 59, 118

N

Navy Bean Soup and Vegetables, 236-37

Neurotransmitters, 302

Niacin (Vitamin B-3)

deficiency of, 116

food sources of, 116

functions of, 116

supplements, 116

Nitrogen balance, 302

Nonheme iron, 302

North, Larry, 95-97

Nutrients

loss of, 112

performance, 174-76

Nutrition, 302

impact on health, 190-92

O

Oat bran, 208
Oatmeal, 208
Obesity, as risk factor for cancer, 145
Oleic acid, 58
Olive oil, 212
Omega-3 fatty acids, 37, 58, 210, 303
Onion Soup, 250
Optimum fueling, calorie needs for,
    189-90
Oriental-type diet, 30
Osteoarthritis, 144
Osteoporosis, 111, 125, 126, 132, 172
    boron in, 129
    and exercise, 150
Oven-Fried Potatoes, 242
Overtraining, 160
Oxalic acid, 125
Oxidation, 193, 212, 291
Oxidative damage, 120-21

P

Pancreas, 46-48
Pantothenic acid, 111
    deficiency of, 116
    food sources of, 116
    function of, 116
Peas
    Minted Peas, 241
    Split Pea Soup, 237
Pectins, 54
Performance nutrients, 174-76

Phenylalanine, 35
Phosphorus, 124
    excess as problem, 172
    food sources of, 37
Phytates, 125
Pinto beans. See Beans
Planned cheats, 188-89, 303
Plantar fasciitis, 176
Pollution, 120
Polysaccharides, 45, 303
Polyunsaturated fat, 303
Pool exercises, 144
Pork, 208
Potassium, 178, 208
    athletic need for, 178
    deficiency of, 127, 178
    depletion, from laxative abuse, 18
    food sources of, 127
    function of, 126-27, 193
    loss of, from self-induced vomiting,
        17
    and sodium, 127, 211
Potatoes, 208
    Baked Potatoes with Tangy
        Toppers, 243
    Egg White Casserole, 219
    Herbed Potato Skins, 242-43
    Mashed Potatoes, 243-44
    Oven-Fried Potatoes, 242
    Potato and Green Bean Salad, 234
    Potato Deviled Eggs, 218
    Potato Salad Vinaigrette, 234-35
    Potato Soup with Chicken, 231-32
    Sauteed New Potatoes, 240

Poultry. *See also* Chicken; Turkey

    white meat, as source of protein, 37

Premenstrual tension (PMS)

    and essential fatty acids, 61

    and exercise, 150-51

Prior, Jerilynn C., 151

ProCarb, 72

Processed carbohydrates, 50-51

Products, recommended, 264-65

Prolactin, 61

Proline, 36

Prostaglandins, 60, 303

Protein, 303

    adverse effects of diets low in,
      30- 34

    and amino acids, 29, 34-37

    animal, 37, 129, 171-72, 213

    complete, 34-36

    deficiency in, 194

    excess as problem, 172

    for exercisers and athletes, 171

    importance of, in diet, 28-29

    and importance of water, 39-40

    on Lean Bodies program, 37-39

    quality, 303

    reasons for need for, 30-34

    sources of, 38

    supplements, 264

    vegetable, 171, 172

Protein powder, 75

Pyroxidine (Vitamin B_6), 36, 178

    athletic need for, 178

    deficiencies of, 117, 151

    food sources of, 117

    function of, 116-17

    supplemental, 117

Q

Quality of life, 195

Quiche

    Spinach Pan Quiche, 259

R

Ratatouille, 255

Recommended Dietary Allowances
    (RDA), 112, 171, 303

Recumbent cycling, 215

Red meat, 39

Repetitive dieting, problems with, 9

Resistance training. *See* Weight
    training

Restaurants, and eating on Lean Bodies
    program, 93-97, 208-9, 283-294

Resting Metabolic Rate (RMR), 23

Rheumatoid arthritis, 144

Riboflavin (Vitamin B-2), 115, 178

    athletic need for, 178

    deficiencies in, 115, 177

    food sources, 115, 177

    function of, 115

Rice

    Beans and Rice Creole, 244-45

    Brown Rice and Mushrooms, 239

Brown Rice Supreme, 238-39

Chicken and Rice Soup, 230-31

Rice and Vegetable Chowder, 235-36

Ringsdorf, Marshall, 4

RNA, 31

Roller-coaster dieting, 206

Rowing, 144

Running, 154-55

S

Safflower oil, 60, 62, 212

  cooking with, 212

Salad dressings

  Basil Vinaigrette, 261-62

  Herb Vinaigrette, 262

  Lean Thousand Island Dressing, 224

  Lemon Mustard Vinaigrette, 249-50

  Potato Salad Vinaigrette, 234-35

  Spicy Vinaigrette, 235

  Tarragon Vinaigrette, 246

  Vegetable French Dressing, 229

Salads

  Asparagus Salad Vinaigrette, 245-46

  Caesar Salad, 248-49

  Fancy Tuna Salad, 224-25

  Gala Cole Slaw, 246-47

  Italian Salad, 248

  Marinated Vegetable Salad, 247

  Shrimp Salad, 223-24

  Southern Salad, 233

  South-of-the-Border Salad, 228-29

Spinach Vinaigrette Salad, 249

Salt. *See* Sodium

Saturated fat, 38, 59, 212, 292

  as culprit in heart disease, 30

Sauces

  Jalapeno Tomato Sauce, 220

  Spicy Salsa, 229-30

Sauteed New Potatoes, 240

Savory Poultry Strips, 227-28

Schaffer, Arnold, 130

Seafood. *See* Fish; Shrimp

Seasoned Fish Fillets with Spinach, 220-21

Selenium, 132

  as antioxidant, 193, 214

  food sources of, 37, 132

  function of, 132

Self-inflicted starvation, 3-4

Semi-vegetarians, 213

Serine, 35

Serotonin, 35

Shrimp

  Barbecued Shrimp, 222

  Shrimp Salad, 223-24

  Shrimp Scampi, 222-23

Simple sugars, 304

Skinfold calipers, 71, 264, 304

Smothered Chicken, 225-26

Sodium, 178, 210-11

  athletic need for, 178

  deficiency of, 178

  and potassium, 127, 211

Soil depletion, 111

Somatomedin, 172

Soups
    Beans and Rice Creole, 244-45
    Chicken and Rice Soup, 230-31
    Chicken Broth, 230
    Navy Bean Soup and Vegetables,
        236-37
    Onion Soup, 250
    Potato Soup with Chicken, 231-32
    Rice and Vegetable Chowder,
        235-36
    Split Pea Soup, 237
    Tomato and Corn Soup, 238
    Tomato Soup, 251
    Turkey and Vegetable Bisque,
        232-33
    Vegetable Gumbo, 258
South-of-the-Border Salad, 228-29
Spaghetti Sauce, 256
Spaghetti Squash, 258
Specific dynamic action (SDA), 32,
    190, 292
Spices and condiments, sources of, 91
Spicy Meat Loaf, 227
Spicy Salsa, 229-30
Spicy Vegetables, 252-53
Spicy Vinaigrette, 235
Spinach, 129
    Seasoned Fish Fillets with Spinach,
        220-21
    Spinach and Mushroom Saute, 259
    Spinach Pan Quiche, 259
    Spinach Vinaigrette Salad, 249
Split Pea Soup, 237
Spotters, 162

Spot toning, 214
Squash
    Spaghetti Squash, 258
    Squash Medley, 260-61
    winter, 50n
    Zucchini and Yellow Squash, 261
Stair climbing machines, 155
Starchy carbohydrates, 48, 49-50, 102,
    304
    exclusion from evening meal in
        Program II, 74-75, 105
    sources of, 90
Starvation, problems with, 5-6
Stationary cycling, 144, 153, 215
Step aerobics, 152-53
Stored fat, 6-7
Stress, 112
    eating under, 213
Subcutaneous fat, 6
Sucrose, 45, 46
Sugars. See also Carbohydrates
    simple, 45-46, 304
Supplemental amino acid growth
    hormone releasers, 181
Sweeteners, 208
Sweet Potatoes with Maple, 245
Swimming, 144, 156

T

Target heart rate (THR), 142
    minimum pace required to achieve,
        157-58

Tarragon Vinaigrette, 246

T-cells, 120, 304

Theophylline, 117

Thermogenesis, 304

Thiamine (Vitamin B-1), 40, 115, 178

athletic need for, 178

deficiency in, 53, 111, 115

food sources, 115

function of, 114-15

Threonine, 35

THR. *See* Target heart rate

Thyroid hormones, side effects of, 17

Tomatoes

Italian Stuffed Tomatoes, 260

Jalapeno Tomato Sauce, 220

Tomato and Corn Soup, 238

Tomato Soup, 251

Trace minerals, 304. *See also* Minerals

Training, meeting nutritional demands of, 181-82

Transferrin, 194

Treadmills, 156-57

Triathlon competition, 171, 178-79

Triglycerides, 47, 146, 304

Tryptophan, 35

Tuna Oriental, 223

Turkey. *See also* Chicken

Savory Poultry Strips, 227-28

as source of protein, 37

South-of-the-Border Salad, 228-29

Spicy Meat Loaf, 227

Turkey and Vegetable Bisque, 232-33

Turkey Chili, 226

Tyrosine, 36

U

Ubiquinone, 134

Ultrasound, 71, 304

Unsaturated fat, 59-60, 304

V

Valine, 35, 180

Vegetables. See also Lean, fibrous vegetables

Asparagus Oriental, 251-52

Asparagus Salad Vinaigrette, 245-46

Beets l'Orange, 252

Broccoli Italiano, 253

Brown Rice and Mushrooms, 239

Brown Rice Supreme, 238-39

Caraway Cabbage, 253

Carrots with Ginger, 254

Cauliflower with Toasted Oats, 254

Eggplant with Spaghetti Sauce, 255-56

Festive Corn, 240

Fiesta Vegetables, 257

Green Beans Italiano, 257

Italian Salad, 248

lean, fibrous, 48, 51-52, 90-91, 300

Marinated Vegetable Salad, 247

Minted Peas, 241

Navy Bean Soup and Vegetables,
    236-37

Ratatouille, 255

Rice and Vegetable Chowder,
    235-36

Seasoned Fish with Spinach, 220-21

Spaghetti Squash, 258

Spicy Vegetables, 252-53

Spinach and Mushroom Saute, 259

Spinach Pan Quiche, 259

Squash Medley, 260-61

Turkey and Vegetable Bisque,
    232-33

Vegetable French Dressing, 229

Vegetable Gumbo, 258

Zucchini and Yellow Squash,
    261-62

Vegetarians on Lean Bodies program,
    213

Vertical climbing, 165

Vinaigrettes

    Asparagus Salad Vinaigrette, 245-46

    Basil Vinaigrette, 261-62

    Herb Vinaigrette, 262

    Lemon Mustard Vinaigrette, 249-50

    Potato Salad Vinaigrette, 234-35

    Spicy Vinaigrette, 235

    Tarragon Vinaigrette, 246

Vitamin(s), 53, 113, 264, 293

    fat-soluble, 113

    need for supplements, 110-13

    storage of, 210

supplements, 113

water-soluble, 113

Vitamin A, 111

    anti-cancer effects of, 114, 192

    as antioxidant, 214

    food sources, 114

    functions of, 113-114

Vitamin B_1 (Thiamine), 40, 115,
    178

    athletic need for, 178

    deficiency in, 53, 115

    food sources, 115

    function of, 114-15

Vitamin B_2 (Vitamin B-2), 115, 178

    athletic need for, 178

    deficiencies in, 115, 177

    food sources, 115, 177

    function of, 115

Vitamin B_3 (Niacin)

    deficiency of, 116

    food sources of, 116

    functions of, 116

    supplements, 116

Vitamin B_6 (pyroxidine), 36, 178

    athletic need for, 178

    deficiencies of, 117, 151

    food sources of, 117

    function of, 116-17

    supplemental, 117

Vitamin B_{12} (Cobalamin), 37, 117-18

    deficiencies, 117-118

    food sources, 37, 38, 117, 118

    functions of, 117-18

Vitamin C, 109, 118-19

anti-cancer effects of, 192

as antioxidant, 193, 214

food sources of, 119

function of, 118-19

Vitamin D

food sources of, 120

function of, 119-120

Vitamin E, 120-21

anti-cancer effects of, 192

as antioxidant, 193, 214

food sources of, 121

functions of, 120-21

Voluntary muscular activity, 190

Vomiting, 17

W

Walking, 141, 144, 157

cardiovascular benefits of vigorous, 146

Water, 209-10

distilled, 39, 211

importance of, 39-40

natural spring, 39

retention of, 33

role of protein in regulating, 32-33

softened, 126

Water-insoluble fiber, 54, 305

Water-soluble fiber, 54, 305

"Weekend Workout" (radio show), 95-97

Weight, definition of, 6

Weight training, 25, 141, 142-43, 214.

See also Exercise; Exercise plan

advanced, 163

and aging, 194-95

benefits from, 143, 146

combining with aerobic exercise, 143-44

reasons for adding to exercise plan, 158-60

safety in, 160-62

Williams, Roger, J., 111

Women

B-complex vitamins for, 178

iron need of, 178

menu plans for, 76-82

minimum pace required to achieve target heart rate, 157-58

nutrient needs of, 111, 125, 126, 129, 132, 150, 172

Workouts, number of, 215

Y

Yogurt, frozen, 208

Yo-yo dieting, 8

link to heart disease, 15

Z

Zinc, 132-33

as antioxidant, 193

athletic need for, 178

deficiency of, 111, 133

food sources of, 37, 178

function of, 132-33, 178

Zucchini

Ratatouille, 255

Zucchini and Yellow Squash, 261